MW01288741

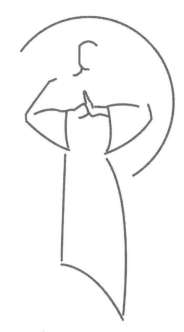

Floating Monk.

The Power of Qigong

A GUIDEBOOK FOR UNDERSTANDING, AND DEVELOPING YOUR CHI ENERGY

To: Elise

For always being a welcome

Face (and warm) hello in every

season   Sifu Jeff

Sifu Jeff Larson

Copyright © 2020 by Sifu Jeff Larson.

ISBN: Softcover   978-1-7960-9817-4
               eBook   978-1-7960-9816-7

All rights reserved. No part of this book may be reproduced or transmitted in
any form or by any means, electronic or mechanical, including photocopying,
recording, or by any information storage and retrieval system, without
permission in writing from the copyright owner.

Any people depicted in stock imagery provided by Getty Images are models, and
such images are being used for illustrative purposes only.
Certain stock imagery © Getty Images.

Print information available on the last page.

Rev. date: 07/03/2020

To order additional copies of this book, contact:
Xlibris
1-888-795-4274
www.Xlibris.com
Orders@Xlibris.com
796548

Contents

Introduction

Sifu Jeff Larson

This book was written for a couple of reasons, first, when teaching this Qigong (and Kung Fu), I found myself repeatedly sharing the history of the System and its Masters with my students. After training with Grand Master Henry Poo Yee, learning about this System, his teacher and the other Masters, I wanted to preserve their names, achievements and the history of this system and it seemed a natural part of a student's training to learn the history of this Art and the insights of the amazing Masters that shaped it.

In addition, one of the most frequent reasons students gave for inconsistent practice was forgetting or confusing the order of the movements, the number of repetitions or some other aspect of the training. In Qigong, as in other physical pursuits, consistent practice is essential to realizing its benefits. Once a student learns to perform the basic movements, they are well on their way to having an effective Qigong program which they can practice for the rest of their life.

Access to our training materials

I have included in this book a list of movements and the order they are done in so that the reader can get a sense of what a basic Qigong program contains. We provide this list of movements, and additional detailed information in all of our Workshops, Private Classes, and Programs of varying length (usually 6-8 weeks).

We are currently redesigning our Website, DVD packaging, Downloads, and other Training Materials. Our website will also provide information about upcoming Workshops, Programs, and access to Private or Semi-Private Classes with our Teachers. In addition, Training Tips, Special Notes, Testimonials, and much more can be found on our site "FloatingMonk.com"

Introduction by Chris Carlson M.D., Surgical Oncologist

Since the advent of Western medicine, especially as it exists today, medical practice has focused its efforts on the treatment of disease. Huge advances in diagnostics and physiology have allowed health practitioners to provide patients with cutting-edge cures for diseases once thought incurable. Examples of the wonders of modern medicine can be found in the eradication of smallpox as a disease, the fact that cancers have been shrunk with multimodal chemotherapeutics, and the use of chimeric antibodies to pinpoint and target specific bacteria.

The achievements and discoveries of Western Medicine and modern medical research have changed and improved our daily lives. From the advent of aspirin to the discovery of penicillin and targeted pain medications, we see evidence of modern medicine's ability to improve our quality of life, including its ability to sustain and even prolong life itself. What Western medicine has lacked, however, is the holistic approach to disease prevention which health practitioners in the East have known about and used successfully for thousands of years.

Since the Yellow Emperor's classic text on internal medicine, written around 2,600 BC and believed to be the origin of Eastern medicine (Traditional Chinese Medicine or TCM), Eastern physicians have studied and mapped energy pathways in the body and learned how stagnation and blockages of this energy can lead to illness. This understanding of the natural harmony of energy pathways in the body has led to a holistic and preventative approach to illness which pervades Eastern culture.

Of all the preventative practices discussed within Eastern medicine, Qigong (pronounced "*chee kung*") is considered to be one of the most powerful and beneficial wellness programs. Qigong enhances our natural breathing process by teaching us to inhale and exhale more efficiently. Some Qigong programs further enhance our breathing patterns by adding relaxed, flowing movements which facilitate healthy energy flow throughout the body along the natural pathways or meridians. These simple Qigong exercises help prevent (and even clear) energy blockages and thus promote health and wellness. The movements themselves are often very simple and easy to perform, so they can be practiced by a person of any age or body type.

As a surgeon and practitioner of Qigong, these two seemingly opposite approaches have made a dramatic impact on my health, my perspective, and how I practice medicine. Qigong practice increases vitality, stimulates the healthy flow of blood throughout the body, and promotes health and wellness. In addition, Qigong uses the body's own physiology to slow the effects of aging, as evidenced in the rosy cheeks and healthy glow of long-time Qigong practitioners.

The simple movements work to naturally fight disease by gently cleansing and oxygenating the internal organs

I believe that Qigong can improve hypertension, decrease the effects of atherosclerosis, and increase blood flow, combating peripheral vascular disease. As one practices Qigong, even for a few minutes each day, you find that you have increased energy throughout the day, that you are able to focus better, and that you experience an overall improved sense of health.

Qigong has not only benefited me physically, the benefit I gain from the quiet, contemplative Moments of my daily practice have made me a better surgeon, husband, and father, and has provided me with a relaxing, enjoyable practice which I will be able to do regardless of my age.

Sifu Larson has been an incredible teacher and inspiration. I have always enjoyed his stories, his sense of history, and the deep well of knowledge he possesses regarding Qigong and its many benefits. I cannot recommend his work highly enough and I encourage everyone to try Qigong for themselves and to experience first-hand the sense of greater health and vitality.

Introduction by Sifu Mark Armstrong, OMD

Please visit "Floating Monk.com" to read Dr Marks captivating Introduction

This book is dedicated to my amazing Teacher and Friend, as well as his Teacher and the other Masters who gave their lives to grow and preserve this System

Grand Master Henry Poo Yee
(Founder of Chinese Kung Fu Academy USA, aka CKFA.com)

Grand Master Lum Sang See
(known as both Lum Wing Fay and Monkey Sang)

Grand Master Chung Yel Chung
(known for both his Medicine Practice and his Kung Fu)

Grand Master Lee Shiem See
(A Taoist Abbot from Wudang Mountain -
Developed Ting Sing Qigong)

Grand Master (Abbot) Som Dot
(Founder of our Art, his Students and Sifu's carried
on his Art until Lee Shiem See arrived)

Chapter 1

(THE PACE AND PRESSURE, AND
THE MASTER'S SECRET)

The pace, pressure, and demands of modern life are affecting our ability to be present and attentive, to just relax, listen, and breathe. The effect of life's hectic pace on us is physical, mental, and in some cases, spiritual. We feel it in our marriages, relationships, and careers. It has us at a point where we're feeling that something has got to change, and we're right.

Individually, and as a society, when we recognize that something isn't working, we attempt to resolve the problem. Sometimes, however, the issues seem too big, or the problems too elusive and we are left not knowing what to do. This feels like one of those times.

Passively and almost unknowingly, we turned away from our intuitive nature, from that quiet voice we used to trust to guide us, the one that rarely lets us down. The noise of life overwhelmed and drowned out our ability to hear that quiet voice and with it our intuitive wisdom. We seem to have lost our compass, doubted, or misplaced our connection to our divine (the divine) and with it the sense of understanding, appreciation, and connection to one another.

Overwhelmed

It has been suggested that people don't care anymore, or that we are either avoiding or unaware of the serious issues. We would rather bury our heads in the sand, in television talent programs, sporting events, and reality shows. Ironically, it's true we are doing that, but it's not because we aren't aware of the serious issues, it's because we are, and at times we're feeling completely overwhelmed.

Something happens when we become overwhelmed; we go looking for ways to convince ourselves that everything is okay, that life is manageable. We begin to reach for happiness in whatever is closest and most convenient. We pacify ourselves with food, numb ourselves with mood-altering substances, and surround ourselves with more material things than we can afford.

It's a natural reaction; food comforts us, alcohol and other substances relieve stress and make us feel better, at least temporarily, and all the stuff we bought helped us convince ourselves that everything was okay, that life was good. There's just one problem. We all know it isn't working, and to compound the problem, as a society we are now overweight, overly dependent on chemical and liquid pick-me-ups, and often deep in debt.

What Now?

The answer is to begin by taking stock of the good within us, rather than beating ourselves up. Our reaction to the intensity of modern life just reminded us that we're human; we were, and still are, trying to convince our families and ourselves that everything is okay, even if we don't believe it. We are just trying to live our lives and be happy.

Solace

We may find some solace in knowing that this has been going on in societies for as far back as we can remember, but there is something very unique about us and this particular point in history. We are the crest of a wave, that point where the wave has reached its peak, just before it folds over and crashes to the shore. Our actions, like the water of that wave spreading out upon the sand, will carry the message of the course we choose and the results which follow.

Destined for Their Time

It has been suggested that certain individuals are born into their time, from ancient times to the modern day. Plato, Aristotle, Benjamin Franklin, Thomas Jefferson, Abraham Lincoln, Ralph Waldo Emerson,

Mahatma Gandhi, Martin Luther King Jr., and even Bill Gates and Steve Jobs all appear to have born into the time that needed them the most.

When the circumstances require it, someone always comes forth with the information that's needed, whether it's to serve a specific need or to advance a society. We believe that the information which we are about to reveal in this book benefits us all individually, and yet also helps us to understand that we are all connected energetically in the dance of life, in our humanity, and this moment in time.

In this book, we provide insight into an ancient practice called Qigong, and share with you information about the Master and the system which he is offering to us. The Master's program can help us turn off the noise of life and the chatter of our own minds and enter into the quiet where we can reconnect with our intuitive self and our innate wisdom. This sounds like something which we can all benefit from, especially now.

Finally, when we consider that the Master in our story is allowing this information to leave the temple for the very first time in history, and that this event is occurring right now in our lifetimes, it seems like more than mere coincidence; it seems almost destined for its time.

Revealing the Master's Secret

In the chapters ahead we take you with us into an ancient world; we will go behind the temple walls where the Masters in our story developed and perfected the secret practices we will share. We will reveal some of the "Unspoken Codes" and tell you how these were preserved and passed down from one century to the next for almost three thousand years.

Until a few years ago, this information was never allowed beyond the temple walls. Even within the temple, access to these secret practices had to be earned through years of rigorous training. Once training in these programs began, learning and assimilating the vast amount of information encapsulated in Qigong took many more years of dedicated practice to complete.

The information we are about to share is one of the most practical and beneficial wellness programs ever developed.

We will share with you the experiences and testimonials of numerous groups and individuals who have learned, and who continue to, practice these programs. We will include our personal stories, the story of the Master, and how these very programs restored his broken body to a state of health and vitality which changed both the course of his life and the history of this system.

With the Master's permission, we are extending our hand and inviting you to join us as we enter a secret world of unspoken codes and ancient traditions. Perhaps upon reading this book, you will share our belief that this ancient wisdom is both applicable and needed in our modern world and in our daily lives.

In earlier times of Temple based training, it is said that once the student had displayed diligent effort for a sufficient amount of the time, that the Master would summons the student to take a walk and to tell the Master why they wish to learn his art. If fortune smiled on the student, the Master may share a special tip or insight to assist with the students learning Sometimes, the student may even be allowed to ask a question of the Master. Such scenarios were referred to as *"taking a Walk with the Master"*

Come with us now and together we will
take – A Walk with The Master.

Chapter 2

"SOMETHING'S HAPPENING HERE"
(A PARADIGM SHIFT)

Buffalo Springfield had it right when they said "Something's Happening Here" in the lyrics of their song about the social conditions of America in 1970. Looking back, life in the 1970's seems much simpler than life in America, and the world, today. Something is happening, and it has only just begun.

In science, when an old view or theory is replaced by a new one (based upon new scientific findings) it is called a paradigm shift. Whenever we enter a new paradigm, it requires a period of adjustment. For example, numerous scientists and academics spend their entire careers validating, teaching, and defending the current paradigm. These theories and principles are understood to be true, until a new paradigm enters their world.

When a new paradigm enters the picture, it is generally met with a great deal of resistance, including repeated attacks to disprove it. The Big Bang theory, evolution, economic anthropology, and even social networking were all new paradigms which met with great resistance. Change, however, is the great constant. Change is ever flowing and unavoidable; we are always changing.

Embracing Change

Generally speaking, we often fear what we do not understand. Change, as a rule, means that we have to adjust to a new situation. We have all experienced this in moving to a new job, a new town, a new school, and so on. Change means that we are on unfamiliar turf, and the unfamiliar is often uncomfortable. At a new job, we are alone among new co-workers. In a new town or school, we have to make new friends.

In our old jobs, towns, and schools we were established and comfortable, now everything is new and uncomfortable.

At present, we are shifting from an old paradigm to a new paradigm; from thinking externally, materially, and often finitely, to thinking, believing, and acting internally, intuitively, and with an awareness of the infinite, and the divine. This is a shift in social and human consciousness. We are all in this together. We are all aware that we were, and continue to be, practically killing ourselves just to keep up, trying to get ahead in the external, materially driven paradigm (the invisible bubble which we are in.) That approach wasn't working, and we knew it intuitively, we just didn't know how to stop it.

We are not going to wake up tomorrow to see that the whole world has suddenly changed. Change, especially internal change, is gradual. What we will begin to realize with greater and greater clarity is that change *has* come. We will find that how we measure the value of our time, our relationships, and even how we expend our energy towards employment has changed. We will begin to notice that the *quality* of our lives is becoming more important and that the *quantity*; the material aspects of our lives is much less important.

We are entering a new paradigm. It isn't something we get to decide whether to participate in or not - the new paradigm has begun.

It should be understood that the material aspect of our lives is not going to go away. We are human. We need certain things to survive and once those needs are met, we will seek to improve our situation, step by step. When we speak of a more aware sense of social consciousness, we are not talking about selling everything we own and running off to live in the woods, although that may be the choice of some people.

An increased sense of awareness or social consciousness begins simply and subtly and expands. It includes looking at your neighbor potting flowers or mowing their lawn and suddenly realizing that we are all here together. It is recognizing that we want many of the same things, and that we are connected in many ways on many levels.

An increase in consciousness sees no separation in life; it does not keep score or seek to get even. We are all part of the whole, the one.

Not everyone will arrive at this awareness at the same time. Those who cling to a world of separation will never have enough, or feel that life is fair, and even. However, every day is a new day, with one more opportunity to walk in the light or to seek and hide in the darkness and negativity. The choice is ours. This book, and the awareness and joy of the Master's Secret, will help us all as we walk in the light and the awareness of our oneness.

In recent years we (in America) have been seeing the influence of other cultures and the ways that they display an appreciation for quality personal time as well as time with family and, perhaps especially, friends. The Swedish Fika, which is the act of taking time alone or with others to pause, enjoy some good coffee or tea with some type of a delicious danish (pastry). In other Scandinavian cultures, such as the Dutch and Norwegians, they have their own version of Fika, called Hygge (pronounced hoo-gah or hue-gah).

The French have always made time for coffees and assorted pastries and while working briefly in England, many years ago, I recall my coworkers asking if we were going to "Have a nice coffee" which meant to pause, exhale and have a break from work and the pressure of our jobs. While traditions like Fika, Hygge, and "Having a nice coffee" are not new to European/Scandinavian cultures, we in America have never had so specific, well defined a moment in our day when we "make time" to stop, relax, enjoy good coffee, fresh pastries, and friendship, perhaps we would do well to adopt such customs.

The Five Thousand Year Cycle

It has been suggested, especially in recent years, that periods of consciousness last for five thousand years. This belief is reflected in the predictions of the Mayan calendar. Some believe that The Mayan calendar embodies a prediction of the end of times or the end of human civilization. This belief is causing a great deal of social dialogue and a considerable amount of fear and stress.

We, at Floating Monk, do not believe that the Mayan calendar speaks about, nor that it is predicting, the end of the human race. The human race has gone through many periods of change over the course of history, and it most surely will go through many more. Change is constant; it occurs within and around us every second of every day. We do believe that through given periods of time there is a prevailing foundational or fundamental consciousness, and that this prevailing consciousness, like scientific paradigms, experiences changes from time to time.

If the changes the Mayan calendar speaks of are related to a shift in foundational consciousness, then we would agree that a shift in social consciousness is either taking root or is already underway. As a society, our perspective is shifting away from an external view focused on separateness toward an internal view focused on our connectedness to everything else within the web of creation; the global community, the eco-sphere, and all life on earth.

With this book, we share with you - the secret programs which a great Master shared with us. These programs are designed to help us turn down, or turn off, both the noise of the external world and the constant chatter of our own minds. When we do this, we enter the quiet where we reconnect with our own intuitive wisdom and feel the presence and the guidance of our personal divine.

This connection is the key to our internal compass; our personal, intuitive, and enlightened guidance system. When we lose this connection, we feel that our efforts do not match the results we hoped for. We feel detached, disconnected, out of balance, and separated. We feel that the energy flow that once guided us and gave us balance is missing.

It is our sincere hope that by sharing the ancient wisdom embodied in the Master's once secret Qigong that your life will be fuller, happier, longer, and filled with greater unity and joy.

Chapter 3

THE MASTER'S STORY - GRAND MASTER HENRY POO YEE (PLUS, THE OPERA SINGER AND MORE)

Born in the United States, Henry Poo Yee went to China to live with his grandmother at a young age. Returning from China to New York's Chinatown at age fifteen, Master Henry Poo Yee's English was extremely limited. With great determination, he graduated from high school, attended college, and completed a BS in Engineering. Building upon his previous experience in the food service industry, he was soon an owner and partner in restaurants and supper clubs. Returning early one morning from New Jersey to New York, Master Yee was involved in a devastating car accident. He was hospitalized for a long period of time, which included considerable physical therapy and rehabilitation.

At the conclusion of his therapy, the doctors arrived at a shocking prognosis. His hand, which was locked in the shape of a claw, was not going to improve. The damage to the muscle and nerves was too severe to expect further improvement; he would have to go through life in this condition. The worst news, however, was still coming. The doctors determined that the circulation to his leg was not going to improve and amputation was required from the knee down.

A few months earlier, the future Master had been a very successful businessman and college graduate with a bright and promising future. In addition to the devastating news from his doctors, other aspects of his life underwent drastic changes while he was hospitalized. The future Master made a bold decision. He checked himself out of the hospital, financially provided for his family, and flew to Taiwan to see his Master, Lum Sang See. Poo Yee had trained with Grand Master Lum Sang See since he was a teenager, around the time Poo Yee entered college Lum Sang See left New York Chinatown and moved to Taiwan. Upon seeing his once promising student arrive at his door, physically crippled and nearly defeated, the Grand Master was moved to tears.

The next morning rehabilitation began. Herbs were gathered from the market; and visits to the nearby country, and a regime of Qigong commenced. At the end of his rehab with Grand Master Lum Sang See, the future Master's hand was relaxed and open and had returned to normal strength. His leg, which the doctors all agreed needed to be amputated below the knee, was also returned to a completely healthy and functioning state.

The Price Tag

Before the Grand Master began treating Poo Yee, his dedicated, long-time student, there was a discussion. If the Grand Master was going to heal his student, he had a request; his student must agree to learn all of the Ting Sing Qigong system. Not only must he agree to learn it, he had to agree to carry it on, teach it and ensure that the secrets were not lost. Poo Yee, the future Master, agreed.

A New Direction in Life

With any decision we make, the direction of our lives may change considerably. The decision to leave New York and travel to seek the assistance of his Sifu was such a decision for the man who is now the Grand Master of our system. A year earlier he was a successful, up-and-coming club and restaurant owner and family man with businesses in New York and New Jersey. Now he was living with his Sifu in Taiwan and had agreed to teach and represent the Master's system. Few of us will ever go through a change that drastic within our own lifetimes.

The Opera Singer

Decades ago, in China, there lived a very successful performer of plays and Chinese Operas. There was, however, a condition which threatened not only her career, but her life; her kidneys were failing. Initially, the problem only showed in one kidney, which she eventually had removed. The remaining kidney appeared to be in good health and her career resumed for a while, but when that kidney began to show signs of trouble, the situation became dire.

The hospital where she had the first kidney removed had done everything, they knew to aid the failing kidney, but nothing worked. She then sought the assistance of hospitals known for alternative natural treatments, but these efforts did not provide the results everyone had hoped for. With her condition deteriorating, it was time to think outside the box. Was there anyone with a non-traditional approach capable of helping her?

Grand Master Lum Sang Sees name came up in these conversations and preparations were made to meet with him. The meeting took place, the terms were agreed to, and the Qigong training began. As a result, her kidney not only returned to its original healthy state, but tests indicated that the kidney was larger and healthier than before it began to fail. In those days in China, it was well known that if someone saved your life, you were committed to serving that person for a number of years out of respect and gratitude.

This famous performer did not want to spend the best years of her career in servitude, so she chose an alternate route, an acceptable course of action at that time; she paid someone to serve as a personal assistant to Grand Master Lum Sang See - in her place.

History Repeats Itself (Sort Of)

In the first six months of the Floating Monk teacher training, Mark Armstrong, OMD, a well-established and highly respected acupuncturist and wellness expert from Atlanta, arrived at his private training class (with me) looking stressed and concerned about something.

I asked if something was on his mind, "Does this system have something to help people with kidney problems?" he asked me. "I have a client who brought her adult daughter to me the other day," he said, "the daughter's skin looked like ash, and she appeared very ill." He then reported that she had just been told by her doctors that she should go home and prepare to die.

She had been on dialysis, but it was no longer helping very much, and her kidneys were very weak. She had been on the list for a transplant but in her current condition was considered too weak to recover from that procedure. I told Dr Mark that our Qigong did have something which may be able to help her; then I told him the story of the opera singer.

I showed Dr Mark the movements most likely to assist this woman, including Chi River Washing, which includes both an internal and an external way to help the body cleanse the kidneys (and other organs) and deliver fresh, more oxygenated blood to those areas. He taught the woman the Qigong which I prescribed. In addition to practicing Qigong, she replaced her old, worn catheter with a new catheter, (the device where the dialysis tubes attach to the body).

Her body responded quickly and positively to the new catheter and the Qigong program which she did at various times throughout the day. She even began to do Qigong movements while she was hooked up to the dialysis machine and asked those around her to respect her silence as she practiced. Previously, it was reported that both the patients and the staff were engaged in unhealthy gossip and loud conversations on a variety of topics that would fill the room for all to hear. In addition, comfort foods like doughnuts and cookies were frequently brought and shared amongst the group.

It has been said that - sometimes it is better to light a single candle than to curse the darkness, and this proved to be profoundly true in this case. What began as a simple request for quiet as she practiced her Qigong, and the dialysis machine filtered her blood, soon became much more. To the notice of staff and patients alike, her condition was steadily improving.

Some of the other patients were now asking if they could sit next to her and copy what she was doing, and she agreed. The loud conversations and the unhealthy gossip which once filled the room steadily faded and were replaced by conversations about getting better, how the patients looked, and felt better than they had weeks and months before. Her doctors, who had sent her home to die just months before, were now suggesting that her condition was so improved they may even take her off the list for kidney recipients.

There is no clear way of determining how great a role the new catheter or Qigong played in her improved condition. All that is known is that her condition improved to a remarkable degree. There is one other element to consider in her improved health and that is her attitude; her faith, her hope, and belief that she was going to get better also played an important role in her marked improvement. Her spiritual faith and the strength she drew from it should also be considered as healing aspects in her journey; from being told to go home and prepare to die, to the vastly improved and hopeful condition which she is in today.

We (at Floating Monk) do not make any claims about Qigong's ability to assist people with serious medical conditions or life-threatening illnesses, but we do stand by the validity, and the truth of the stories we share with you. Furthermore, we are very careful to ensure that any statement we make is backed by research, is something we have experienced or witnessed first-hand, or comes from a source we know and consider to be above reproach.

Chapter 4

UNDERSTANDING CHI (THE ORIGINS OF QIGONG AND THE TWO SCHOOLS)

Qigong, (pronounced *chee kung*) is also called Chi Kung in North America and many European countries. There are additional ways of writing or pronouncing Qigong, but the meaning is the same; they all refer to breathing practices which are often credited with improving health, increasing our life energy and life expectancy, as well as promoting the healing of ailments or injuries. As a general rule, Qigong programs are done either sitting or standing and often include a series of gentle, flowing movements.

The Translation of the word Qigong is this: (*qi* or *chi*) means "breath" and *gong* (or *kung*) means "work." These words also have a deeper meaning: *chi* means energy or life force, and *gong* (or *kung*) means an advanced training practice.

Qigong practice may also be described as:
A method for understanding, developing, and
manifesting your life energy - Chi

The reason there are so many stories about Qigong achieving amazing results is that Qigong deals directly with your life force, your chi. By using your breath, body postures, and gentle, flowing movements perfected over many centuries, these programs circulate your life force, your chi, throughout your body. As your chi circulates, it removes blockages allowing your energy, your life force, to flow properly. The next step is to increase and store even more chi and then learn to focus this energy towards your goals and visions for life. The results and benefits are as varied as the programs being offered. For this reason, it is important to verify the credentials of both the program and the instructor. Read more on this in the section "The Unspoken Codes."

Where the Secrets Began

Prior to sharing the Master's gift, it is important to have at least a basic understanding of where Qigong comes from, how it evolved, and why this Master's information remained a secret for all these years. We will provide the following brief history of Qigong prior to discussing the Master's secret. Later in the book, we will provide a more detailed history of the Master's System, including how he formed the first new branch from the original system. We will also explain how Floating Monk followed the Master's example and became the first, and to date only, new branch from his lineage.

In the Beginning: The Ancient Caves

The earliest records of Qigong date back about six thousand years to caves along the Yangtze (also known as the Yellow) River in China. On the walls of these caves were drawings of bodies performing what appear to be an interconnected and flowing series of movements similar to the movements used in Qigong. There is no information available about these drawings, yet experts suggest they are the earliest known depictions of Qigong.

The Yellow Emperor: The Birth of Traditional Chinese Medicine (TCM) and Qigong

The most conclusive documented information on Qigong takes us back to the time of the Yellow Emperor Huangdi. The period of The Yellow Emperor in China extends from 2,697 to 2,597 BC. The Yellow Emperor is credited with the formal introduction of Traditional Chinese Medicine, as well as the first recorded material on Qigong. As the record indicates, the Yellow Emperor lived to over 100 years of age.

From the Two Schools to the World

Generally speaking, after the time of The Yellow Emperor, Qigong practices developed and grew forth from two different sources or schools: Taoist and Buddhist (Shaolin). The Taoist temples produced numerous Qigong programs as well as the popular exercise and Martial Art known as Tai Chi. Likewise; the Buddhist (Shaolin) temples also produced many powerful Qigong programs but are more readily known for bringing us Kung Fu.

Northern and Southern China

Martial arts and Qigong systems often define themselves as being Northern or Southern, meaning from Northern or Southern China. The movements of the Northern systems tend to be wide and sweeping and take more room to perform. The Southern systems tend to have shorter, more compact motions and favor close-range fighting or contact. Geography helps us to understand the reason for this as the North has sweeping plains and more open spaces, while the South is characterized by bamboo forests and more confined terrain. Taoist systems are often viewed as Northern (especially from the Wudang Mountains, in the Wudang Region, and Buddhist (Shaolin) systems as Southern, although this is by no means a hard and fast rule.

Our Programs

The programs we are about to share with you operate from a fundamental belief that all of us have a personal life force, or personal energy. This energy, for over three thousand years, has been called Chi. Our programs teach you to move this energy, or Chi, throughout your body to reduce stress, relax your mind and body, enhance your circulation, cleanse and strengthen your internal organs (your engine) and provide you with more energy than you've probably felt for many, many years. Our programs also go beyond teaching you to move your natural, given Chi, we will address this in the pages ahead.

Qigong as Medicine

For thousands of years, specialized breathing programs were one of the primary tools of Traditional Chinese Medicine. These specialized breathing programs were developed over the course of many centuries. Many Shaolin and Taoist monks dedicated their entire lives to developing and perfecting these programs. These specialized programs were referred to as Qigong and those who perfected these systems were known as Qigong Masters.

The Fountain of Youth

Over the centuries Qigong has been referred to in many ways: the fountain of youth, the breath of life, the secret elixir, the practice of the three treasures, prana, and many, many other names. Certain, advanced Qigong programs, teach practitioners to make their bodies conduits between Earth and Heaven by first drawing the energy into themselves, and then releasing the energy back to its source.

Some of these programs have been preserved over the centuries, some have been lost to time, and others, like the Qigong in this book, had never been allowed to leave the temple, remaining a secret for all these years.

Their Secret Weapon: Chi

The specialized breathing programs (Qigong programs) developed and practiced in ancient Chinese temples have slowly come to public knowledge over the course of many centuries. For time immemorial, it has been rumored that the monks in these temples, and many of the legendary warriors in Chinese folklore, had developed special powers through the practice of Qigong, in other words, *that Qigong was somehow their secret weapon.*

The Master: Passing on the System

In this book we explain to the reader a set of simple, yet very unique programs which can increase energy, advance awareness, improve health, and perhaps even prolong life. These secret programs were passed down from a great Master to his inner circle of long-time disciples called the Enter the Gate Disciples.

> *The fact that Grand Master Yee is allowing us to share this gift with the public at a time when it is so needed is more than a simple gesture of kindness It is an Act of Love.*

Our Thoughts and Our Energy

Wherever we direct our thoughts and our attention, we are also directing our energy. Our thoughts are energy and the actions we take are expressions of that energy. We intuitively understand this when we say, "I have a lot of energy today" or "the energy in the room was really good." This idea, which seems profound, is actually something we not only understand, but refer to throughout our day. When quantum physics proclaimed that "Everything is Energy" it didn't come as news to us, we (as a Collective Society, and as Qigong students) already knew this.

The simple daily programs we present in this book, which appear to be a new way of approaching and energizing your day, are not new at all; these programs are the pearls of ancient wisdom. These enjoyable, easy-to-perform programs of relaxed breathing and gentle movement that help to increase, store, and manifest our energy date back thousands of years. They have been practiced, preserved, and passed down from one Master to the next this entire time.

Energy: the Alpha and the Omega

We use the word energy frequently throughout this book, primarily as it refers to "your energy," the energy within you, and the universal energy that surrounds you. The programs, which we will reveal and discuss, will tell you how to increase, store, and manifest your energy towards the powerful and attainable vision you have for your life.

With the Master's permission, we are inviting you to join us as we enter a secret world of unspoken codes and Ancient Traditions.

This Ancient Wisdom is both applicable and needed in our Modern World, and our daily lives. Journey with us through the chapters ahead as together, we take . . .
A walk with the Master

Chapter 5

UNDERSTANDING A PAI

Both Halves of the Circle

As we pull back the curtain and begin to reveal the structure, practices, and principles of the ancient temples, we first need to tell you what a Pai is. This understanding will give you the ability to look at any program and accurately define whether the program is a Pai, a Style, or simply information that was gathered and put together to develop a specific type of Program.

For me, as a long-time practitioner of a very traditional temple-based system, I ardently believe in teachers being up-front, honest, and willing to share with students the origins, history, and validity of any program they are offering.

As Qigong grows in popularity, which it will for many years to come, there are those in our society who will see Qigong as an opportunity to enrich themselves and will rush into the public square with programs which may, or may not have true histories or, provide real value.

In short be alert and always seek a good, truly Certified Teacher because, ...

The Charlatans are coming!

There are few things that disturb us (true Martial Artist) more than dishonesty. If someone has dedicated themselves to a noble and true practice, put in the time, worked hard, and learned a program, then by all means they have earned the right to represent that program in the public arena.

We firmly hold that every program being offered to the public should meet specific criteria. The minimum requirement should be to clearly define the source of the information, such as we have done by providing the history of our program and identifying every Master up to the present day. We also believe that adherence to the Unspoken Codes is part of this requirement as it asks the question; "Who's Your Sifu?" and allows the student to determine if the Sifu (teacher) Reflects the Light.

In traditional Qigong the teacher (Sifu) is a messenger, a reflection of the light (The System and the previous Masters). The Sifu is a reflection of the original system and the Master's that came before them. When the role of a teacher is viewed in this way, it is extremely important that the teacher's actions honor the linage of their system.

A Pai, a System, or a Program

In the Qigong (and Kung Fu) world there two main descriptors: 1) a complete System or Pai, and 2) a Style. In the past few decades, a third term has emerged: a Program.

A Pai refers to a Complete System. A complete system has two halves, like the two halves of a circle. One half is made up of forms, fighting, and weapons; the other half is medicine, healing, and Qigong. The Master of a Pai often excels in other areas as well, such as calligraphy, philosophy, poetry, painting and other such disciplines which we in Western civilization often refer to as "the Arts and Letters."

These two halves serve to balance each other. If you learn to kill, you must learn to heal. If you learn to strike, you must learn to yield. If you condition your bones to be like steel, you must also be able to flow like water. The symbol of yin and yang (aka yum/yang), the balance between both halves, is symbolic of a complete System or Pai. In order to have a Pai, it is necessary to have a Master. We do not mean someone who has mastered a Style or a Practice, we mean the Master of an entire System.

A Style is not a complete System; a Style reflects pieces of a complete system. As a general rule, a Style is designed specifically for fighting. A style does not teach a complete program, it is a piece of a program, or a piece of a Pai. *Many of the martial arts schools in North America and Europe today are Styles.*

In ancient times there was no such thing as a police force. In those days the wealthy families in towns and villages, and occasionally the villagers themselves, paid accomplished martial artists to teach them self-defense. This was accurately depicted in the movie *The Seven Samurai.* These martial artists taught the townspeople and villagers the easiest, most direct and lethal techniques they knew, including open hand and weapons techniques, which they gleaned from the martial arts system they had trained in. Many of the Styles which are popular today actually originated in this way.

A **Program is neither a Pai** (a complete system) **nor a Style** (a piece of a complete system). *Programs are often developed using pieces of information from a variety of sources.* At other times, programs were developed using a single idea or practice from a Pai, a Style, or even from another program.

Numerous self-help programs, as well as many modern practitioners using titles like energy worker, energy healer, and energy guide and other such titles *do not provide any specific, historical source as the foundation of their training, understanding, or skill.*

Others claim to have information from, or a connection to, a wide variety of sources. Having information from a wide variety of sources can be a good thing, but we believe that the practitioner offering services to the public owes it to them to identify those sources as well as the level of understanding, training, and certification they have achieved.

The American Indian culture is an excellent example of identifying the source of their knowledge and the level of their understanding. In the American Indian culture, the practitioner, Shaman, or Medicine Man (or Medicine Woman) always identifies their tribe, their teacher, and their level of understanding. This kind of openness and honesty not only respects the source of their knowledge as well as the Grandfathers and the Great Spirit, it also demonstrates a respect for the person coming to them for treatment or healing.

Identifying the source and showing a respect for the system, the teacher, the tribe, and the culture is of vital importance. It is this acknowledgement which helps to create the connection to the spirits,

Great Spirit (American Indian) or the Masters and the Universe (Chinese) whose help, energy, and guidance the healer is seeking to transfer to the person who has come to them.

We prefer to believe that every individual, and all of the groups that are currently offering services in the public marketplace, are sincere in their efforts and that their intentions are good. As for our organization, we know what we offer, and we speak about what we know. It is not our place to speak to the validity of other programs, but we would offer this piece of advice: the Unspoken Codes can be applied to any program, and the answers you receive should provide the information you need to make an informed decision.

Math and Mystery

In the ancient temples, Qigong programs were developed and perfected within the framework of a complete system or Pai. As we mentioned, a Pai is symbolized by a circle, with two equal and perfectly balanced halves. Balance was the objective; life was the journey or the process.

From the early days of mathematics, pi symbolized as ϖ (equaling 3.14159) is a mathematical constant that is the ratio of a circle's circumference. Because the definition of pi relates to the circle, pi is found in many disciplines such as trigonometry, geometry, mechanics, and electromagnetism. The further one advances into Qigong (and the martial arts) the more you see and understand the theory and application of geometry and physics. With enough time, you will come to see movement in terms of geometric or mathematical shapes and formulas. *Like the circle, the further you get from the source, the closer you get to the beginning.*

In the later, more advanced stages of Qigong practice, quantum physics becomes more and more relevant, especially in describing what is happening in terms of energy. *This may sound complex, but it isn't, it is as logical as it is simple.* As Quantum Physic states: "Everything is Energy." When energy is blocked, we feel uncomfortable, frustrated and out of balance. When energy is flowing, we feel light, energetic and in balance. We as a society use expressions like this every day, so the discussion of energy is not foreign to us at all. We just didn't realize how clever we were, *we have been talking in terms of quantum physics our entire lives.*

Ancient and Modern

From Ancient Greece we received the formula pi "ϖ," and from ancient China we received the term Pai, represented by the yin-yang symbol. Both pi and Pai refer to circles, both are constants; they are unwavering. Both of these symbols serve as foundations. Pi "ϖ" serves as a foundation for mathematics, mechanics, engineering and more. Pai, represented by yin/yang, serves as the foundation for balance of two separate yet equal and united halves. It speaks to the idea of spirit and body, of internal and external (or inside and outside), of upper and lower, and of body and mind.

Encapsulated within the symbol of yin-yang is the idea we refer to as: As Above – So Below. This idea is interwoven into any definition or explanation of the two halves of the circle. The symbol of yin-yang and the concept of As Above-So Below permeate all of human existence. They serve not only as guidelines for practices within systems; they provide a philosophical foundation for what we do, and how we live our lives. Finally, both symbols remain as relevant today, in the twenty-first century, as they were the moment, they were first conceived. Grand Master Yee spoke extensively about the concept of "As Above - As Below, as students of this System of Qigong - you shall grow intimately well versed in the both theory and practice of this idea, and it will amaze you!

Qigong is not Tai Chi

Publicly, there is confusion regarding Qigong and Tai Chi, namely that people often think they refer to the same thing. They do not.

Tai Chi, known formally as Tai Chi Chuan, is a Martial Art System. It is a product of the Taoist temples or the Taoist school. Tai Chi Chuan means Supreme Ultimate Fist. Tai Chi is widely known as a gentle, slow-moving exercise, which we often see being practiced in public parks, especially early in the mornings.

In reality, *Tai Chi Chuan is an extremely powerful and highly effective Martial Art.* There are a number of excellent Tai Chi Masters in the United States and Canada who teach Tai Chi to the full extent of its potential, but there are also a number of teachers who teach Tai Chi as more of a gentle exercise than as a powerful martial art.

Tai Chi Chuan as a system (or Pai) does have numerous Qigong programs, many of which are referred to by animal names or as various treasures. These Qigong programs vary widely depending upon the teacher or Master, including the range of the programs which they know (have trained in) and/or are willing to teach. Perhaps the biggest reason that Qigong and Tai Chi are confused by many people is because they sound similar; both Tai Chi and Qigong have the word (word sound): Chi in them.

Summary

There are many different types of Tai Chi, as well as numerous different systems of martial arts, and many of these programs offer their own unique type of Qigong. The fact that there are so many diverse programs to choose from makes it very difficult for someone to know which to choose.

Keep it Simple

At Floating Monk, we believe that programs should be clear, easy to explain, enjoyable to perform, and that the benefits should be felt as early as the first class. We also believe that it is vital to be honest with oneself about how long you are willing to practice each day. The majority of our programs are designed as ten to fifteen-minute practices, but they can be performed as longer practices. If a person is rushed on any given day, or simple prefers a very brief practice, they can do a simple five-minute program. On days when a person has more time, they can do twenty minutes or more, adding the Stretching Qigong to the Sitting or Standing Qigong for an even more enjoyable and beneficial program is always an option.

A Note regarding other Programs and Styles of learning

We want to pause for a moment and step back from the Micro (more intricate) view of Qigong which we are discussing in this book and remind the reader that there are many styles of Qigong. This book speaks to the Ting Sing Qigong shared with us by our teacher Grand Master Henry Poo Yee and referred to as Floating Monk (and Chi for Health) Qigong we teach publicly today. There are literally hundreds of Qigong programs in the world today. Each Martial Arts program which is a Pai is likely to have its own, unique Qigong program.

As interested individuals, it falls to us (meaning those seeking to be students) to research the marketplace, read about or go to watch various Martial arts and Qigong programs and then decide what approach we are most interested in or believe we would enjoy the most and perhaps gain the most from.

Chapter 6

THE MASTER'S SYSTEM IS A PAI (П)

The Master we refer to in this book is Grand Master Henry Poo Yee. Great Grand Master Lum Sang See (his teacher) gave Grand Master Yee the nick name Poo (or Po) in reference to the Last Emperor of China, Po Yi. Perhaps Great Grand Master Lum Sang See had a vision of the legacy which Grand Master Yee would create and gave him this nickname as a reference to what he would accomplish and the impact his knowledge would have upon the world. It is our understanding that when Poo Yee was learning from Master Lum Sang See in New York Chinatown, in his youth, That Lum Sang (also known as Lum Wing Fay or Monkey Sang), had sole possession of the name *Kwongsai Jook Lum Gee Tong Long Pai, also referred to simply as Jook Lum Gee Tong Long Pai in the U.S.*

The original Kung Fu system in which *Ting Sing Qigong* originated is called *Kwongsai Jook Lum Gee Tong Long Pai.* As indicated by its name, it is a complete system, or Pai. From its origin in the 1800s, prominent names associated with the system are Som Dot, Lee Shiem See, Cheung Yel Chung, Lum Sang See, and the current (recently deceased) Grand Master Henry Poo Yee. For detailed information on these Masters, as well as more information about the System, visit Grand Master Yee's website CKFA.com and click on History. While you are there, be sure to click on the tab for Grand Master Yee's personal history, we are confident that you will enjoy learning even more about him.

Grand Master Yee forms a New Pai

When Grand Master Yee completed his rehabilitation with Great Grand Master Lum Sang See and accepted the responsibilities associated with his new title, he decided to form a new branch from the original tree. This new branch would be the very first Pai born out of the original system. Grand Master Yee named this new Pai: Chinese Kung Fu Academy U.S.A. (CKFA.com). This information is also available on the Grand Master's website. Please understand that this information is greatly consolidated for reference here, also understand that we (the author) seeks to be respectful to all parties involved in this discussion of history and the systems name.

Grand Master Yee would tell us, his students, that in the years following Master Monkeys move to Taiwan, a group of dedicated, long time students (in New York Chinatown) affiliated with the original school requested the rights to the Pai's name. Master Yee said it was agreed that they would hold title to the name and help to preserve the system from their organization in New York, NY. We came to understand that this action also played a part in Master Yee choosing to call his new Pai: Chinese Kung Fu Academy USA or CKFA for short. Although Master Yee's Pai held a different name now, the history of the system, as a branch from the original tree, remained the same.

Preserving CKFA and the Houston Headquarters School

Many years before his passing, Grand Master Yee put in place a process of Annual Student Reunions and other ceremonies so that when he passed there would be no misunderstanding of who he had chosen to maintain and preserve the system he created. In the years just before he passed, he set in place a group of individuals to carry on his teachings and continue the Headquarters School he established in Houston, TX. In addition to regular training classes, and various outreach programs, the school is continuing the Grand Masters practice of having an Annual Student Reunion of all the Branch Schools each year. The Annual Student Reunion was previously held in November (recently moved to February-March). To attend and train at the reunion, or to inquire about classes contact the Headquarters School at CKFA.com

The Lead Instructors, who are charged with carrying on the CKFA Headquarters School and CKFA as an Organization are: Sifu Tommy M Quan, Sifu Paul Dermody, and Sifu Abraham Chu.

(Sifu Sapir Tal) runs the program in Israel and longtime advanced Sifu's such as Bruce Campbell and Paul Huber remain active as respected mentors within the organization. In addition to the Headquarters schools there are many highly qualified Sifu's throughout the US, Canada, and Israel, see list below:

Headquarters School		713 779 1089
	Sifu Tommy Quan	832 860 8878
	Sifu Paul Dermody	832 303 2532
	Sifu Abraham Chu	832 878 6988
Boston, MA	Sifu Khanh Ly	617 733 1417
Atlanta, GA	Sifu Peter Goulbourne	404 309 9889
	Instructor Jonathan Gass	678 908 3233
	Instructor John Hall Jr	678 371 5481
St Louis, MO	Sifu Peter Scheers	314 484 0507
Ventura, CA	Sifu Alfanso Silinas	805 240 1286
Camarillo, CA	Sifu Eddie Urbistondo	805 384 2378
Malibu, CA	Sifu Eddie Urbistondo	805 384 2378
Habal Shem Tov 47	Sifu Sapir Tal	
Petah-Tikva, Israel	sifusapir@gmail.com	Int + 972-52-2508570

Floating Monk is born

When Grand Master Yee allowed me to take the Qigong out of the temple and teach it to the public for the first time, he made his permission conditional. The name Ting Sing could not be used in the public arena, it had to stay in the temple.

For the first few years, I called the Qigong Chi for Health, a name I still really like and use for certain programs, many people still know it by this name, but Internet searches revealed that this name may be too generic - I did not want people attempting to find us via the Internet to get lost in a sea of chi-related queries, so a new name was created to stand alongside Chi for Health.

In Chinese mythology (see the book trilogy called "Outlaws of The Marsh") there were a group of very unique messengers with secret talents. These messengers were called upon whenever important information needed to get to the Emperor, or between generals who were some distance from one another during great battles and at times of war. It was rumored that these messengers would write special symbols on pieces of paper, adhere the paper to their calves, and that upon doing so they would levitate.

Using the power of their intent, it is said that these monks could travel at great speeds and that if seen from a distance they appeared to be floating. These monks were aptly referred to as The Floating Monks. We believe that we too are the bearers of important information, because we are bringing the information about this unique Qigong (Grand Master Yee's Qigong) to the public for the first time. It is for this reason that we chose to call our organization Floating Monk and named the Qigong: Floating Monk Qigong.

I spent many years asking Grand Master Yee for permission to teach this Qigong to the public before he finally relented and gave me permission. Perhaps my constant pestering played a part in Grand Master Yee finally saying Yes, and allowing me to teach this Qigong publicly, but I believe it was actually the Master's observation of the condition of the world in its present state, and the need people have for the kind of benefits which this Qigong provides.

The Alter

When Grand Master Yee finally gave me permission to teach this Qigong It was not simply a great honor, this was a historic event. In the entire history of this system, no one had even shown the movements of Ting Sing Chi Kung beyond the temple walls. This is a responsibility that I (now we) do not take lightly. We strive each day to provide students with the same high-quality training and discussions that our great teacher, Grand Master Henry Poo Yee shared with us. To validate this moment and to display to the world his approval of this event as well as my position as his dedicated, long time student, Master Yee did something else which (to my knowledge) he had not done before, nor since, he presented we with an Alter.

To those who understand the significance of this act, no additional words or information are needed. To those who do not know the significance of this act, no words of explanation would be sufficient. Being presented with an alter and informed about (some of) the rituals which are required to maintain the alter, is one of the highest honors a Kung Fu student can hope to experience.

Many years later, after visiting China on more than one occasion, Grand Master Yee become very discomforted with a story he heard about one of the Masters of the system during the second World War. This story was later proven to be false, but by then (regarding my alter) the damage had already been done. During this period of unease (between trips to China as memory serves) Grand Master Yee was removing anything around him which bore this Masters name, this also meant speaking with me, about the alter, either at a Student Reunion or during a Summer Private Training Session, I do not recall which it was.

Jeffries, Sifu said, Sifu always called me Jeffries (versus Jeff, Jeffery, etc.) I want to talk with you about something. Sifu told me the story he had heard about one of the Masters in our system, he shared why he was so unsettled and then he presented me with a dilemma. Sifu said; you can keep the alter and follow your own path, or you can burn the alter and follow me. I chose option number two. Instructions were given for a certain month, on a certain day and a specific time of day to carry out the task. I was also given specific instructions as to direction, i.e. North South, East, West and I agreed to burn the alter according to the instructions given

This was a task I knew I must do but it was such an honor to receive the alter that burning it tore at my heart. I carried out the task as instructed, specific date, time, direction, etc. I phoned Sifu the next day to inform him that it was done. After I told him I was silent, he too said little and our conversation soon came to a close. Yes, there is proof of the Alter, I took pictures with students before that alter on the occasion of certain training accomplishments on their part. Regarding the Master whose name was smeared, in a subsequent trip to China, Sifu came across new information, as well as physical proof that the previous story was false, the Masters name was cleared of any unfitting action. As a result, the alter did not need to be burned after all. Perhaps there are other, unknown, or additional reasons for burning the alter, if so, I do not know, none of us will ever know.

Chapter 7

BASIC MOVEMENTS OF QIGONG (A GUIDE)

Student Handbook: Standing Chi Kung - Level I

Floating Monk has a variety of unique and interesting programs. The common thread that runs through all of the programs is a firm understanding of breathing, motion and energy.

In this program you will practice simple up and down motions and learn to connect your breath to your motion. We are confident that you will fell lighter and more energized the "very first time" you try it.

The Standing Chi Kung is the cornerstone of the Floating Monk Qigong System. Each of the Qigong Programs offers a great deal of benefit, but the Standing Chi Kung is the most powerful

Standing Qigong

- **Take your place on the Earth** (the 6 steps)
- **Breath normally for a few breaths**
- **Bend knees, lower body, release tension**
- **Knees & elbows / lift the torso / elbows back**
- **Chop wood / shoulders forward, breath to chest / bend knees**
- **The pacing breath**
- **Yin / Yang / Yin**
- **Close**
- **Body washing - brushing**
- **Shake out / Twisting**
- **Salute to Close**

Student Handbook: Sitting Qigong - Level I

Floating Monk has a variety of unique and interesting programs. The common thread that runs through all of the programs is a firm understanding of breathing, motion and energy.

You will learn many things, including: Yin/ Yang/ Yin, *The Four Chimneys, Chi River washing, the Four Exits, and much more.* Once learned, you can perform the Sitting Chi Kung in as little as 8 to 10 minutes and begin to experience for yourself the benefits of Floating Monk Sitting Qigong.

Sitting Qigong

- **Sit forward on a chair** (a non-metal chair preferably)
- **Sit with knees aligned inside shoulders**
- **Palms in cup position / elbows out/ palms to Heaven**
- **Breathing: 12 Yin / 2 Yang / 1 Yin**
- **Closing**
- **Chi River Washing**
- **Stand up – shake out**
- **Twisting**
- **Walk the circle**
- **Salute to Close**

Our Programs

Our system contains three specific Qigong platforms, they are: Sitting Qigong, Standing Qigong, and Stretching Qigong. The information within these programs is divided into the following levels:

Sitting Qigong Levels, I and II
Stretching Qigong Levels, I and II
Standing Qigong Levels, I, II, III, IV, V (level V is the highest Sifu level)

How You Benefit:

Sitting Qigong

To the casual observer unfamiliar with Qigong, it would appear that a person doing Sitting Qigong is sitting still doing very little. The first part is true, they are sitting fairly still, although there is some movement, but the thought that they are doing very little would be completely incorrect.

Bruce Lee referred to meditation and Qigong type programs as: Active Inactivity. From the outside it appears that very little is happening, while inside a great deal is happening. This effectively describes Floating Monk Sitting Qigong. The Sitting Qigong program is wonderful for people of any age. It is also an excellent program for businesses and organizations as it can be done in work attire.

Sitting Qigong is also very popular with those who have injured joints, muscles, or other health issues which make it uncomfortable to do the Standing Qigong. Medical and Rehabilitation Facilities, Wellness Centers, and Senior Activity Centers also tend to favor the Sitting Qigong Program.

A Truly Unique Program

No other program uses the same sitting posture, hand and arm positions, and breathing techniques as Floating Monk Qigong. The information we provide about the flow of the breath, the movement of the Chi through the body, the change in hand positions, and the transition from Yin to Yang and back to Yin provides a clear, practical, and easy to follow series of movements, allowing even a first-time practitioner to enjoy and benefit from our programs.

In the first class alone, many students said they learned more than they had at the completion of other programs. After we guide beginning students into the proper body posture, we explain what the posture is designed to do, and how. We inform students about what they may experience and then we begin the practice of Sitting Qigong.

Standing Qigong

The Standing Qigong program is the central program of both Floating Monk and the original Ting Sing Qigong System. The Floating Monk Standing Qigong program has three main levels; each level is needed due the vast amount of information and technique in the complete program. The longer you train in Floating Monk, the more you come to understand and appreciate the depth of the knowledge, as well as the logic and practicality, behind each and every movement.

> *One of the most appreciated aspects of Floating Monk Qigong is that it builds upon the information and techniques of the previous levels.*

> *This varies significantly from many Qigong programs - which teach a new series of motions with every level.*

In the beginning program, we teach practitioners how Chi moves through the body in a circle. The Level I program introduces the idea of circular breathing, as well as the up and down movements, and explains how the movement coordinates with the breath to create a powerful sense of flowing energy throughout the body.

Level II Standing Qigong introduces what we call the Six Sections of the Circle. Practitioners then learn how to move various groups of muscles in coordination with the breath. This smooth, relaxed, synchronized movement creates an even more powerful Qigong experience.

Levels III, IV, and V

The most unique and powerful movements of the Floating Monk Qigong program are found in these levels. Level III and above are for individuals who want to experience Qigong in a way that they may not have previously imagined. We reserve the right to teach these levels to those who are serious about Qigong, especially those interested in teaching and helping us to bring the benefits of Floating Monk Qigong to more people.

How Much Qigong is Enough?

The first two levels of Floating Monk Qigong are the foundation for the higher levels. Understanding and effectively practicing the first two levels provides a vast amount of benefit to the practitioner, so the higher levels are not a necessity. If someone is truly determined to learn the higher levels, or they are committed to learning and teaching the first two levels of the program in partnership with Floating Monk, it is best to practice Levels I and II for some months (even years) before proceeding to the higher levels.

> **Grand Master Yee was very fond of telling**
> **students regarding the first two levels:**
> **"If you learn this Qigong, and you practice regularly**
> **you have enough Qigong for the rest of your life."**

Stretching Qigong

The Sitting Qigong and the Standing Qigong are a direct reflection of the Ting Sing Qigong from which it originates. The Stretching Qigong encapsulates principles of the Ting Sing, but also information gleaned from Shaolin Kung Fu training and other related programs over more than thirty years.

One of the primary goals of the Stretching Qigong program is to teach the practitioner how to use the breath to have a conversation with the body. The timing of the inhale and the exhale are coordinated to specific movements. Many long-time practitioners of other stretching and breathing programs have told us how much they appreciate the logic and organized flow of movements within this program.

The Series of Movements

The Stretching Qigong program warms and "oils" every joint in the body. The program begins with a twisting technique popular in Taoist internal cleansing programs. Once the body is warm, the Big Circles are next, followed by a stretch called Greet the Day. The next series stretches warms the large muscle groups in the front and back of the body, followed by long, relaxed side body stretches.

Once the series of stretches is complete, a series called The World of Circles follows, then the Windmill, sideways Windmill, and chest and back stretches with a few twists near the finish. The final movements of the Stretching Qigong are front and back leg stretches, followed by a few additional twists to complete the program and prepare you to meet the day.

Health from the Inside Out

Perhaps the best way to understand health from the inside out is to consider what it means to be healthy. Good health and overall vitality are predicated on all of the organs of the body working well independently - and in unison - with one another. Have you ever seen an ad for a fitness program with talked about the health of your organs? The fact that you probably haven't underlies how health and wellness is perceived in Western culture.

In the West

In the West, many exercise advertisements show people in their early twenties to their early thirties wearing spandex and looking ripped as they jump, pump, bend, and sweat. There is nothing wrong with being physically fit, looking good, and feeling good about it. That's not the point. Congratulations to those who do such programs and enjoy them. The point is that Western exercise is often focused externally while the focus of Eastern wellness and fitness programs is from the inside out.

In the West, appearance is supreme. Fitness is frequently measured in terms of appearance; looking and acting young is favored over age, experience, and wisdom. Traditional Chinese medicine states that energy must be balanced and in a state of flow for an organism (or individual) to function properly and to flourish.

In the East

From an Eastern perspective, health is viewed much more from the inside out. In the East, evidence of good health is measured by clear skin and eyes, energy, vitality, and even by obtaining old age. Those who live well, exercise (which often includes Qigong), and achieve a healthy appearance and old age are revered, and their advice is sought by those who respect their age and wisdom.

It is neither fair nor wise to make bold claims, to say that one way is good and the other is bad. In the measurement of wellness, as in life, the truth is often somewhere in between. We understand and appreciate the benefits of Qigong and believe that a person of any age will feel better, healthier, and have more energy by practicing Qigong, but we also recognize that everyone must find their own way.

Ponce de Leon and the Search for the Fountain of Youth

When the Spanish explorer Ponce de Leon embarked on his famous voyages in search of the fountain of youth, he went looking externally, whereas he may have had better fortune by looking within. He may also have benefited from interviewing those who possessed the gift of health and old age, and considered what they were doing internally, such as their diet, rather than focusing completely on a mythical spring which contained the secret of eternal youth.

Chapter 8

BEHIND THE CURTAIN (THE SECRET TECHNIQUES REVEALED)

Grand Master Yee has spent his life training, perfecting, preserving and passing on the Kung Fu of the Chinese Kung Fu Academy U.S.A. and the Ting Sing Qigong which Great Grand Master Lum Sang See taught him.

Without Grand Master Yee's permission, this Qigong would never have been available to the public, and the lives of many people who have benefited from this Qigong would be very different. In addition to our gratitude to Grand Master Yee, we are also thankful to his Sifu, Great Grand Master Lum Sang See, and Great, Great Grand Master Lee Shiem See for developing the original program.

Mensa meets Shaolin and the Tao (A Master like No Other)

The impact that Great, Great Grand Master Lee Shiem See had upon this system was, and remains today, immense. His level of intelligence is displayed in his understanding of the *I Ching* (The Book of Changes), Taoism, Buddhism, Astronomy, Physics, Geometry, Electromagnetism, Chinese Medicine, Nature and the Four Seasons, and much more. The great Master brought his understanding of all of these areas together in one place, the Qigong Program which he developed and titled Ting Sing Qigong.

Ting Sing means "To make the Universal Shine." In application, this means to make the energy of the universe shine forth from you, the practitioner. In all the years of training and teaching Qigong and Kung Fu, through local, state, regional and national/international tournaments, observing numerous Master's demonstrations, watching film, and reading a wide array of books and assorted research, I (personally)

have never seen a Qigong Program that is anything like Lee Shiem See's
Ting Sing Qigong.

Immediate Benefit

One of the most intriguing aspects of Ting Sing (Floating Monk
Qigong) is that the benefits begin as soon as you start to practice.
Of course, the more you practice and the better you get at relaxing,
breathing, and performing the movements - the more benefit you receive.
The movements of this Qigong are simple and easy to understand, and
this simplicity allows students to adjust or correct their posture when
practicing on their own.

When the teacher tells you what these simple movements and
breathing techniques are doing, and you feel the Chi inside your body
wake up and begin to flow, you start to really enjoy, understand and
connect with the Qigong. Once this happens, which is usually very
early in Qigong training, *you begin to look forward to waking up and
practicing your Qigong every day.*

A Glimpse inside the Qigong

A simple list of some of the elements which Lee Shiem See includes
in this Qigong will help to clarify the depth of his wisdom:

- Stepping Into the Circle
- The Four Directions
- The Two Vortexes
- Finding your Place on the Earth
- The Six Sections of the Circle
- As Above-So Below
- The Three Rings of Chi
- The Four Winds
- The Four Chimneys
- The Four Exits
- Eating from Heaven

- Yin/Yang/Yin
- The Three Gates
- Thunder in the Cave
- The Highest High
- The Empty Force
- The Five Elements
- Washing The Chi River
- Reverse Breathing
- The Zipper
- Opening and Closing the Third Eye

*It wasn't a matter of just being incredibly intelligent
Great Grand Master Lee Shiem See was a Genius.*

Stepping Into the Circle

Stepping into the Circle is the technique which begins the Qigong practice. There is a visual component related to this technique, and from the very first moment on the very first day, this technique lays the foundation for something we call: The Conversation with Heaven. Once inside the circle, you begin to adjust your feet; this is the beginning of the Four Directions, which leads to the Twin Vortexes and Finding Your Place on the Earth. This technique is only practiced with the Standing Qigong.

The Three Treasures

The Three Treasures is not an idea unique to Floating Monk; it is part of a broader philosophy. According to Taoist doctrine, the Three Treasures can be described as the three types of energy available to humans. Speaking generally, they are known as Jing, Chi, and Shen.

Jing refers to our human bodies and its abilities. Chi refers to our personal internal energy and our life force. It is important to note that Chi is considered to be in all things.

Shen refers to the spirit. Within this context it refers not only to our spirit, for it presupposes that we have a spirit, but to the broader spiritual world beyond and above us. In some Qigong practices it is believed that the practitioner may enter Shen.

The Twin Vortexes

To begin Floating Monk (Standing) Qigong, the practitioner steps Into the Circle, adjust the feet in a prescribed fashion, and begins to circle (rotate the body). To the casual observer, this motion looks very odd, but the Floating Monk practitioner understands this motion is creating what we call the Twin Vortexes. The first vortex draws the energy from the earth upward into the body. The second vortex draws the energy through the body and sends the energy toward heaven, from which it returns.

The more familiar and more comfortable the practitioner gets with this motion; the easier it is to relax and thus flow within the motion. The footwork, including the width of the feet and the movement within the feet, requires that they be positioned correctly. The motions must be properly performed to create the desired effect.

The Four Winds

The Four Winds element introduces itself very early in the Standing Qigong and arises again with greater detail in the more advanced practice. The Four Winds is very prevalent in Level III and Level IV. It refers not only to the four directions, but also to the angle of the hands and arms while performing the movement.

When practicing the Four Winds, if the angles of the hands are correct, the hands will adjust the wrist, the wrist will adjust the elbow, the elbow will adjust the shoulders, and the shoulders will speak to and adjust the body. The entire body will be one, which is flowing with and connected to the energy and movement. If the angles of the wrist are not correct, every other section of the structure will be, what we refer to as, broken. If the structure is broken, the energy will not accumulate or run properly throughout the body.

Yin/Yang/Yin

Yin/Yang/Yin is one of the most profound and yet easily understood concepts of our practice. Yin/Yang/Yin, loosely translated, means soft/hard/soft. The introduction of this theory places us firmly on the doorstep of quantum physics, there's simply no way around it. We mentioned earlier in the book that everything is energy. It is here in Yin/Yang/Yin that the presence of quantum physics becomes clear.

In both Standing and Sitting Qigong, most of the program is done in a relaxed (yin) state. At a specific point towards the end of the exercise (in Sitting Qigong) the practitioner adjusts their hand position in preparation for squeezing the body which is a transition into yang. The practitioner will apply a squeezing motion at a specific point in the breathing cycle and will perform this yang technique for a specific number of cycles. Following this series of yang squeezes, the practitioner transitions briefly back into a yin state. This practice is known as Yin/Yang/Yin.

Opening and Closing the Physical and Energy Body

When the practitioner is in the yin state, muscles, bones, and tendons are relaxed. *The idea is for this relaxation to reach all the way down to the cells of your body.* This relaxation allows for the free flow of the energy inside the body. When the body is sufficiently yin (open) the entire body begins to breathe in the air and energy around it. When you transition in yang, you learn to seal in the energy that has entered your body. Upon return to a yin state, you do what we call scanning the body, which sends the mind and breath through the body to search for, speak to, and relax any muscle or organ that might still be tense, or what we call *holding*.

As Above-So Below

As Above-So Below is a broad idea that refers to matching, repeating, mirroring, and at the same time balancing, that which is on earth with that which is in heaven. It also refers to the upper half and the lower halves of the body.

We mentioned in Yin/Yang/Yin that there were points in the form where you squeeze the body. Applying this concept to the concept of As Above-So Below (in the Standing Qigong) if we squeeze at a given point when the hands are in the upper part of the body, then we must also squeeze when the hands are located at a given point in the lower part of the body.

The Four Chimneys

The Four Chimneys refer to four locations on the body. During the practice of either the Sitting or Standing Qigong, the body creates heat. In the body's effort to disperse or release this heat, it uses the Four Chimneys, which we also refer to as vents.

As the body disperses the heat through these vents, it carries some degree of moisture along with the heat, which we refer to as steam. It is believed that this steam carries with it the impurities that are present in the body. For this reason, we say that as the body releases this steam out of the Four Chimneys, the body is steaming out the poison.

New Qigong practitioners are very often surprised to find that a measurable amount of steam has been released by the body through the Four Chimneys, and yet they did not feel it (or sometimes believe it) until they checked the locations of the Four Chimneys and realized that it had occurred.

Internal and External

It may seem odd to mention the word "external" in the context of describing a Qigong program, after all, isn't Qigong an internal practice? The answer to that question is both yes and no. Yes, Qigong is considered an internal exercise or program because it is primarily a practice of specialized, relaxed breathing techniques; however, there is an external aspect of Qigong as well: the skin.

We often refer to Qigong as a program of health from the inside out, meaning that it focuses on breathing and the health and vitality of the internal organs. Many people are surprised, however, when they are asked to name the largest organ of the body - it is our skin. That's right, our skin is an organ and it is the largest organ of our entire body.

A Complete System and a Complete Qigong

Earlier, we defined what a complete system, or Pai, is. Not only are there complete systems in martial arts, there are complete systems in Qigong as well. A complete system in Qigong, as symbolized by the yin-yang symbol, has two parts: internal and external. Sometimes, although it is quite rare, a system may have (as Floating Monk does) a Yin/Yang/Yin component as well.

Washing the Chi River

The external component of Floating Monk Qigong is called: Washing the Chi River. Between (and within) each of the seven layers of skin, and between the skin and our muscles, is a fluid, referred to in Qigong as the Chi River. The Chi River, it is suggested, becomes polluted with toxins as the body works to filter itself and maintain proper balance.

Chi River Washing uses a special series of techniques to rid the body of the toxins within. This process also helps to reduce naturally occurring stress hormones, such as cortisol. Stress hormones can build up and cause our body's considerable stress-related damage, including heart attacks and stroke. *It is important when reviewing various Qigong programs to know if they have a process for Chi River Washing. Simply speaking, in most cases, they will not.*

The Four Exits

In the process of external cleansing such as washing the Chi River, it is important to consider how the toxins and other impurities are going to get out of the body. This leads to the discussion of the Four Exits.

Actually, there are a total of six exits, but the first four are specifically related to the Chi River. It is not enough for a program to suggest that a process or technique helps to cleanse the body; this is the information age and we want to know exactly how the program actually does what it says it can.

Of all the aspects of various Qigong Programs, I am most surprised, and disappointed, when I learn that a practice not only does not have a process that relates to the Four Exits, but also has no knowledge of them. I simply cannot fathom this idea and practice not being central to any Qigong practice. However, we must accept that - there are a hundred roads to Rome! Also, many Qigong practices may have very valid reasons for the ideas and the movements they perform.

Chapter 9

THE MASTER'S SECRET (HEALTH FROM THE INSIDE OUT)

In the pages leading up to this chapter, we have mentioned a number of benefits related to the practice of Floating Monk Qigong. It is now time to talk specifically about the Master's secret.

The Master's Secret, The Master's Gift is - This Ancient Qigong

Qigong's Biggest Secret

Throughout this book we explain why Qigong, Floating Monk Qigong (aka Chi for Health) in particular, is so beneficial. We describe how Qigong improves circulation, enhances metabolism, and oxygenates the body. We also describe how the gentle, flowing movements of Floating Monk Qigong warm and strengthen the joints and tone the body.

Traditional Chinese medicine prescribes Qigong for the treatment of numerous maladies. Hospitals in China have been incorporating Qigong into treatment programs for many years. In addition to the testimonials of Qigong practitioners, research into Qigong, going on for decades, shows overwhelmingly positive results. Yet for all of the evidence related to the benefits of practicing Qigong, there is rarely a whisper about Qigong's biggest secret.

Qigong's biggest secret has long been known by advanced practitioners, Sifu's, and Masters, but it is rarely discussed publicly. It is rooted in the understanding or belief that there are two types of Chi. The first type of Chi is referred to as natural Chi, or simply Life Force, this kind is also referred to as Innate Chi. This is the Life energy or Chi you were born with. It is believed that we are all born with a certain amount of life force, some believe that that once this supply is used up, it is gone forever. The second type of Chi is referred to as Acquired Chi and, as the name implies, this Chi is acquired from an outside source.

Simply stated, and by this I mean I will save you a decade of research with no conclusive result, and go directly to the concluding statement: *The only means by which a person can obtain additional life force (Chi) is believed to be through Qigong.* This - is Qigong's biggest secret. In high-level Qigong circles, this belief is considered to be a truth, and evidence of this truth is found (primarily but not exclusively) in the long lives and healthy physical condition of Qigong Masters, as well as in the healing powers of certain Qigong practices.

Generally speaking, Qigong Masters and Sifu's are not interested in challenging the principles they hold to be truths. Truths are self-evident; they are supported by the principles, practices, and simple logic of the Qigong programs. Further, Qigong teachers have the benefit experiencing the benefits for themselves as well as seeing the benefits in their students.

These Qigong truths are also closely held beliefs which Sifu's and Masters are not interested in laying bare for public scrutiny or clinical scientific examinations, and double-blind studies by earth bound and physical reality-based scientist intent on debunking their beliefs. *This is one of the reasons why Qigong's biggest secret is rarely, if ever, discussed.* The idea that Qigong can (possibly) help a practitioner obtain additional life force (by acquiring Chi energy from the universe that surrounds us) is what makes it unique from all other practices.

We firmly believe in the benefits of a variety of physical activities, from gardening to running, biking to yoga, walking, weight-lighting, boxing, or any array of cardiovascular and strengthening programs. In fact, many of these types of programs offer physical benefits that Qigong does not.

One may well enjoy many forms of physical activity, and wisely so, but we believe that the addition of Qigong will largely prove to produce positive results and a fuller, healthier life. Qigong is one of many options for improving health and prolonging life, but in our view, Qigong is unique in its approach to connecting with and enhancing our internal life force, or Chi.

Ting Sing Qigong

Ting Sing Qigong is the name of the Qigong related to this specific Pai (K*wong Sai Jook Lum Gee Tong Long Pai*). The name Ting Sing remains inside the temple. We use the name Floating Monk when showing and teaching this Qigong to the public. As I mentioned previously, in Chinese mythology the Floating Monks were known as the messengers of important information and we felt this name was fitting because we (as an organization) are bringing this valuable information to the public for the very first time.

A Hundred Roads to Rome

We use the word Rome as a metaphor for a goal, a destination, or a place a person is seeking to reach physically, philosophically, or even spiritually. When teaching Qigong, we explain that there are a hundred roads to Rome. Rome (the destination) may represent peace of mind, a sense of calm, or a feeling of spiritual connection. It can also be a feeling of connection to our intuitive wisdom or our personal divine, which awaits us all - *inside the quiet.*

You do not need to choose to practice Qigong over practicing some other program; perhaps one of the best approaches is to combine Qigong with activities you already do, especially as Qigong practice can be done in increments of a few minutes, or as a complete exercise in fifteen to twenty or thirty minutes. Qigong works wonderfully in conjunction with other more physically demanding activities.

Choosing the Road That's Right for You

The very next section will describe how the Floating Monk Qigong programs can help you to live a fuller, healthier, happier, and more energetic life. We sincerely hope that you find our programs of value and that you make a little time to enjoy them daily. If you choose another road or another program for your current path, we hope that you will enjoy it and find it fulfilling. Should you ever choose to train our programs in the future, our doors are always open, and our dedicated instructors remain ever willing to teach you all that they know.

Chapter 10

THE UNSPOKEN CODES

The Unspoken Codes

Behind the temple walls, steeped in ancient tradition, are the Unspoken Codes. These codes have guided the behavior of Qigong Sifu's and Masters from the earliest days and are as alive today as they were thousands of years ago. When Teachers, Sifu's and Masters bring their knowledge to the public arena, other Teachers, Sifu's and Masters are watching to see if they are following the codes.

The Inner Circle

Membership in the inner circles of high-level Qigong is steeped in ritual; burning incense, kneeling, saluting, recitations, and a number of other aspects which unfortunately cannot be mentioned here. The details of what occurs during these ceremonies are not what's important, what is important is the commitment to uphold and reflect the integrity of the system, both publicly and privately.

These commitments encapsulate what we refer to as the Codes of Conduct. The uniqueness of the Codes of Conduct is that, in many cases, these codes are embedded into the information provided and the terms which are agreed to, but they are not verbalized. *These commitments exist as a type of contract. If you walk a certain path you are expected to abide by this unwritten contract; you are expected to uphold the codes.*

The codes are the guidelines for the Sifu's behavior, especially in public, and you never break the codes.

The codes are the links of a chain that connects the Sifu to those that came before him or her, and you never, ever break the chain.

What are the Secret Codes?

It is an unwritten rule that the codes are expected to be maintained by each system that offers its programs to the public, and by the individuals who represent that system. There is no established group for monitoring the codes; they are the guidelines by which a Sifu is to monitor their own behavior. Invisible to the public eye, these codes are the lens through which Instructors, Sifu's and Masters observe the public behavior of their peers.

These codes are referred to, almost in passing, during the ceremony, marking your entry into the Inner Gate. In a strange and mysterious way, the fact that some of the codes are mentioned so subtly actually punctuates their importance. When the Master casually talks about what can occur if certain codes are broken, *you suddenly realize that the stories and mysteries which you have heard about and wondered about for so many years are actually true.* That realization is a powerful and memorable Moment.

The Codes which May be Mentioned

Of all the rules within the codes, there are a few which may be mentioned publicly because they deal with public behavior. In the coming years, as Qigong becomes more and more popular, we believe that it will be beneficial for the public to have some way of understanding and differentiating between various types of programs, including those that do and those that do not follow the codes.

Of the codes which may be mentioned
The First is known as   **"Reflecting the Light"**
The Second is   **"Who's your Sifu?"**

The First Code: Reflecting the Light

There is a belief in Chinese culture regarding success, it says: "Be careful about rising - too high or too fast - because the higher you go, the further you can fall."

This idea does not suggest that a person should not try to be successful; rather, it speaks to the idea of being sure-footed, and of building on a sound foundation. Success can be fleeting, or it can be long-lasting, and the definition of success varies between individuals, cultures, and nations.

This idea is reflected in Western Culture, and this is most often referenced in success in Business and in Motion Pictures, it says: Be careful who you step on - on the way Up - because you will see them again on the way Down."

In Qigong, we believe that success begins by giving credit to those responsible for it, including recognizing, naming, and showing gratitude towards that person. Success in Qigong means Reflecting the Light. An ancient tradition, it is one of the most fundamental Unspoken Codes.

Historically, it would have been applied the first time that a Master graduated a student and allowed him or her to go out into the world to begin their teaching career. Every time that new teacher received praise, the next words out of his or her mouth should be *"thank you, I had a Great Teacher.*

Humility

At the center of Reflecting the Light is humility. True humility is sincere and grateful; it recognizes that your success is owed in part (often in large part) to the time and energy that your teacher has dedicated to you, and the information (often once highly secret information) which they have imparted to you. Yes, you had to do the work, often a great deal of work once you possessed the knowledge, but still, your teacher had to give it to you.

We see reflections of this code within our own society, for example, when a public figure or celebrity speaks about how a certain teacher influenced their life. They tell stories about how a certain teacher or college professor saw something in them gave them their time and guided them, this - is Reflecting the Light. The same principle holds true in Qigong.

There is something innately satisfying about being in the presence of someone who is truly great and sincerely humble. Mahatma Gandhi and Martin Luther King, Jr. were such individuals. Other such (secular) persons may include Albert Einstein, Ralph Waldo Emerson, Robert Frost, numerous Amazing Film Directors, The Roosevelts, The Kennedy's, T. S. Eliot, Mark Twain, and Quincy Jones. As a society, we tend to have great respect for those who show sincere humility, and in like fashion we tend to abhor those whose egos far exceed their talents or their deeds.

The Codes as Guides

The Codes of Conduct are there to provide a guideline which we can use to see who is Reflecting the Light, and they help to steer us clear of those who Absorb the Light. In Qigong, someone who Reflects the Light always happily gives credit to their Instructor, Sifu, or Master.

When you compliment someone who Reflects the Light, the very next words out of their mouth are always, "Thank you, I had Great Teacher." Likewise, someone who Absorbs the Light will take the credit, mention nothing of their teacher, and wear their knowledge (or fame) publicly with arrogance and pride.

The Second Code: Who's Your Sifu?

In their entirety, the Codes of Conduct speak to behavior both public and private. Individuals who follow the path the codes outline are inwardly focused on their own behavior; they don't teach the codes (that is the role of each instructor's Teacher or Master) or admonish anyone who lives by other guidelines. *They simply live their lives by quiet example.*

The codes will not be found anywhere in writing. They are never mentioned in the literature about classes, workshops, or in any training manuals. The codes are rarely even discussed outside of the special ceremonies where a Sifu or Master is graduating a student. If you have the opportunity to train with a Certified Sifu, you may hear them discuss behavior in general terms from time to time. The onus is on the student to pick up on these subtle suggestions for they are the Sifu's way of giving the student insight into the Unspoken Codes.

Behind the curtain, however, in the world of Certified Instructors, Sifu's, and Masters, these codes are considered unwritten law. When a teacher introduces themselves, whether it is to another teacher or to a class or workshop, the introduction should always be: "Hello, my name is (their name), I teach (the name of the system) and my Sifu/Master is (Sifu/Master's name)." This script should never, ever vary!

The Question Has Three Parts

For someone who is seeking out a Qigong program to study, the codes provide these simple questions. To the question of, who's your Sifu, there are three parts that, added together, will provide enough information to let you know if you are speaking with a Qualified, Certified Instructor who follows the codes and Reflects the Light. The three questions are:

The Three Questions:

What System do you Teach?

Who is your Sifu / Master?

What level are you Certified to? As a Teacher?

At first glance

At first glance these three questions seem really, really simple, and they are. However, experience is a valuable teacher and it shows us that even those who claim to be Masters, in some cases, never even trained

Qigong specifically and if they did - never did so with a Master or, were never certified as Instructors.

Others, say they trained with a Chinese Master, or one or more Teachers / Masters (usually in China they say) - yet they never name the Master / Teacher, never provide evidence that the stated Master is in fact a Master/Teacher, never name the System, never provide the History, the Linage, *the Level or verified Instructor status of those they say they trained with or evidence of their own achievement of Instructor status.*

This is a really, really serious issue in Chinese & Martial Arts Culture, a student always, always, always says who their Master was, what the System was, when they trained (how long) or what level they trained to - failure to do so is Highly, Highly Questionable!

Others - never say where they trained (such as Province, Town, Temple)

- never say how long they trained for (from date x to date y)
- never say what level they trained to
- never say if they were Certified as a Teacher / Sifu
- never produce evidence of their Certification

A new System / Qigong practice

Is it possible, or allowed, or has it been known to happen that an accomplished Martial Artist creates a new program, piecing it together form one (or many) arts they have trained? Yes, absolutely, and there is nothing inherently wrong with such an act – as long as – the Teacher states what they have done.

If, however, one practices an Art - which does not have Qigong in its practices – and then claims Qigong Teacher status, or moreover "Mastery" (or being the Master) of a newly named Qigong, this…is highly suspect and potential students may wish to travel further down the road to a school with a true linage, one where the masters are known by name and date, where the linage is clear, the certification is verified, and all other aspects (listed above) are also presented openly and without request.

Chapter 11

FROM ORAL HISTORY TO WRITTEN TEXT - THE JOURNEY (TRAINING MANUALS, DVDS, DOWNLOADS)

Traditions

Traditions, once established, remain as they are until someone changes them. In the world of Qigong, and much of martial arts, traditions are in many cases, hundreds, and in some cases, thousands of years old. One of the oldest traditions in the Qigong and Kung Fu world relates to passing on the secrets of a system from generation to generation, from one Master to the next.

In most cases, written information of some kind passes from one Master to the next, but in many cases, the Masters are the only ones who will ever see this information. Only recently have programs begun to produce written information. Even in recent times, programs will advertise publicly and provide brochures (with a brief bio of the Master/Instructor) when you visit the school, but that would often be the last time you would see anything about the system in print.

Most of the instruction in traditional schools is oral, from the history of the system, to the programs offered, to the levels within the programs. The programs themselves, including every movement in every form, is passed from teacher to student orally. This was the tradition and it was never questioned. If you did talk about it privately with your classmates, you never considered asking the Master why more of the information was not in written form.

An Entire System

Imagine for a moment what it would be like to write out each and every movement of a form that took just a minute or two to perform. It may not sound too difficult, but as soon as you begin describing every hand, elbow, shoulder, waist, ankle, and knee motion for a single set of movements, you soon realize that the task is far bigger and much more laborious than you had initially imagined. It is almost an impossible task.

In addition to the motion itself, now consider explaining what the breath is doing, and what the muscles are doing, besides the movement. Now add the intent, where your mind is focused (or not focused) while you are performing each technique and suddenly you begin to understand the scope of such an undertaking.

This is one of the reasons that so little of the information on Qigong and Kung Fu programs is written down. If a program is generous enough to write out what it offers and provides some information about the levels within the program, you should consider yourself fortunate.

Student Notebooks

Much of the specific information about various forms, and the nuances within the forms, can only be found in two places; the first place is in the Master's mind and the second place is within the pages of the student's notebooks. We were sometimes allowed to break away during our training to make notes about a new form or a particular technique. At other times, especially when the Master was talking, we knew better than to even ask. At those times we did our very best to listen closely, knowing we would make our notes later.

Teaching is Learning

It has often been said that the best way to learn something is to teach it. I firmly believe in this approach. No matter how well you think you know something, you will never be sure until the moment you try to teach it. When you have to explain the order of a particular series of motions, and begin to take questions or provide explanations regarding why something is done, or not done, a particular way, you begin to appreciate what it means to truly know something well.

In teaching, you must revisit everything you have ever learned about the given subject. You go back and study your notes, and you mentally review what it was like when you were trying to learn a form or technique for the first time. You find that you have to think deeper; you think through what a form or a technique is trying to accomplish, and you realize that you have to know the entire system far more intimately than before.

You begin to realize that you cannot merely *teach Qigong*, you have to *become Qigong*. That is where the journey truly begins. You probably won't realize it at the time, but once you start down that path, you will never return as the same person you were when the journey began.

Ting Sing Qigong had an Oral History

When the Master gave permission to take this Qigong out into the world, allowing it to be shown to the public for the first time, it existed entirely in oral history. There was not a single word related to any technique or form written down anywhere, except in student notebooks. In addition, the system had been taught layer by layer over a period of many years, and during this time additional techniques were added to specific sections, there were techniques that were alternates for other techniques, and so on.

This Qigong had always been taught as part of a Kung Fu system, and then only to the serious, long-term practitioners or students of the Master. The Qigong was totally separate and unique from Kung Fu, but we were used to learning this way, getting little pieces of information over a period of many years. The way that we had learned Qigong was unique; it was not a process that could be used in teaching to the Qigong to the public - An entirely new approach had to be developed.

Initial Efforts

I had already been teaching Qigong to Kung Fu students for many years. We were always allowed to teach the Qigong as a part of Kung Fu, but, with the Master's recent permission, I would now be teaching Qigong as a separate program. Martial arts instructors – whom I had known for many years, as well as friends and relatives of my Private Students, became my first students.

I monitored the results as I taught, watching for progress week by week. I soon realized what I considered to be an error in the way that I was teaching. I was teaching the program in much the same way that I had learned and was practicing it, and that was the error. When I began to learn Qigong, I had already been training Kung Fu for many years, so I understood the terminology, and the movements came almost naturally to me.

These new students did not have such references, so the amount of information I was giving them was both too extensive and too advanced. I realized that I would have to dissect the entire program and rebuild it, piece by piece. I concluded that, once the fundamentals were in place, the students would have a foundation and I would be able to slowly add new information.

Beginning at Square One

I began by categorizing the programs into Sitting, Standing, and Stretching Qigong. The process of breaking down and recording all of the techniques, for each of the programs, took a very long time, but it was absolutely essential to do it this way. The Master had given me the Qigong, often in complete sections, over many years, now I had to determine where the line was between one level and the next.

Initially, I structured the information into three levels, but the amount of information on each level was still too great, the amount of information was over-whelming my students and the process of learning even the first level took far too long.

I had to go back and dissect the information again, to make each level less arduous and more enjoyable to learn. Once this task was complete, years after the first efforts had begun, the process was complete; there were now five levels (to become a Black Sash Sifu), and that is the way the program remains structured to this day.

Chapter 12

TURNING THE LIGHT TO THE HEART

Many years ago (while living in Atlanta), I was asked to come to Augusta, Georgia to teach a workshop for a group of Physical and Mental therapists. The sponsor was a physical therapist who owned and operated two clinics and had been on the faculty of the Medical College of Georgia, a prestigious school located in Augusta. The group consisted of doctors and accomplished practitioners in the mental health and physical therapy fields, among others.

On my drive from Atlanta to Augusta I had been considering what this group of professionals needed to hear that was different than any other workshop or group of students. As I walked into the room (saluted and introduced myself) and sat down facing the group, I sensed that there was an air of anticipation. I looked out at the group and one of the first things I told them was this:

> *"If you practice this Qigong program, you should prepare yourself because one of the effects of this practice is that it turns the light to your heart."*

Whatever your current beliefs are – they will grow strong

What I was trying to prepare them for was that the program they were about to learn would begin with what we call "turning off the noise." When you turn down or turn off the noise of life and chatter of your mind, you slowly enter into the quiet. You then, naturally, begin to ask yourself what is really important. This noise-free environment shifts the light (the attention) away from the chatter of your mind and toward those things which your heart truly desires – and believes in.

Once this idea began to sink in amongst the crowd, I continued: "If you like the work you are doing, then you will love this Qigong because your inner-self is about to steer the light in that direction. If, however, you do not like what you are doing, if you are questioning your passion, or perhaps are unsure where your passion truly lies, you will be made aware of it as a result of this training.

It is amazing what your heart will reveal to you when you turn your attention away from the daily chatter of your mind and toward your heart, meaning toward what you really (honestly) love, enjoy, or want to do with your life.

If we were to replace the word "heart" with the word "soul" or "spirit," what we are saying here would take on a much deeper meaning. As you read and re-read this section about turning the light to your heart, consider the idea of soul or spirit and you may gain additional insight. We are using the term "light to your heart" because this is the way it is taught, however, as many of us know, Eastern philosophies often present ideas using terms and symbols which are easily understood or easy to relate to, but the idea, like an onion, may have many layers.

This same effect holds true for relationships. One of the things practitioners find when they begin our programs is a conscious awareness of what they value. This frequently evolves into an awareness of what they most value in their relationships, with their work, with their spouse or partner, and elsewhere in their lives.

When we think about it, we often find ourselves saying: Of course, it's so simple, why did I not see that before? One reason, though there are many, that we may never have consciously considered this before is because we were trying so hard to be happy. Suddenly we see it (In our minds eye) and it all seems perfectly reasonable and clear.

In our view, we are spiritual beings living in physical bodies. Naturally, we want to be happy, to meet and even exceed the necessities of physical existence (through our homes, jobs, cars, clothes, food, and other material items) *but as spirits we know there is more to our current existence.*

Qigong, while being an incredibly beneficial physical practice,
is also one of many roads to greater spiritual awareness.

When we watch a theatrical play, we see what is occurring on the stage in front of the curtain, but if they were to pull back the curtain, we would see that there is a lot more going on than what we originally observed. Our programs are much like a stage play in this way; the practice is like the scene upon the stage, but the result, the experience, and the journey are similar to what occurs behind the curtain.

In our programs we use the term "conversation" quite frequently. In the Stretching Qigong program, we talk about your breath having "a conversation" with your body. In Standing and Sitting Qigong, we talk about the conversation between your breath, your muscles, and your mind. On the first day of the first program, we talk about finding your place on the earth, and as the programs advance, we talk about "the conversation between Earth and Heaven". The word Heaven could be switched with the word cosmos, the conversation would still be the same.

Chi: Our Life Force

The energy that flows through the postures of the Qigong begins within our bodies; it is the energy of Chi; our life force. Soon after learning how to circulate your own energy, we discuss drawing in and releasing the energy that surrounds you through the air we breathe. In time, we discuss the energy of earth and heaven, *and how your body is a focal point and a conduit between the two.*

Recognizing, nourishing, and participating in this flow of energy is what we call "the conversation." As the conversation becomes more active, through attentive practice, the energy expands. When this occurs, the energy goes outward and upward. Over time, your sense of awareness, intuition, and connection becomes stronger.

The Path toward Love

At Floating Monk, we neither teach nor profess any specific philosophical or religious belief, in part, because the very process of practicing these programs will lead you to your own insights. Also, it has been our experience that whatever spiritual faith you hold within you, whatever source you consider your divine will become clearer and stronger as a result of entering into a conversation with the energy within, around, and beyond you.

We believe that every faith, life view, and philosophy will eventually meet on one central path, and that – is the path towards Love.

Grand Master Yee taught us this

Chapter 13

THE STORY OF THE BENDING HOUSE
(A TRUE QIGONG TALE)

The thoughts of Sifu Tony Fabriguze
Written by Sifu Jeff Larson

I have always loved incredible stories of superhuman strength, tales of unusual powers, visions of martial arts Masters leaping onto rooftops or dropping from great heights. These were, in part, the types of wonder-filled, mysterious visions and abilities that initially drew me to Martial Arts training. I admit, I doubted that these tales were true, but honestly, I wanted them to be, and part of me held out belief they could be. I wanted to believe in the things I'd seen in movies like "Crouching Tiger, Hidden Dragon" and the "House of Flying Daggers" among others and thought surely somewhere there are martial artists with skills like that - there must be. In my mind there was a martial arts story to match the Charles Atlas tale of the skinny kid on the back cover of comic books who morphs into the strong, muscled-up defender of not only of skinny kids like himself, but of defenseless people everywhere.

As kids, we all wanted to be the Saturday afternoon western movie guy in the white hat. The good guy, the lone force between good and evil in the world. This was, and is, the underlying current that drives many martial artists, and that was certainly a part of what drove me to train. Over time, as I shared these ideas—these visions, hopes and dreams with other martial artists, I came to learn that we all love the tales of mystical powers and super strengths, but most of us doubted that we would ever witness such feats, moreover, that we would possess such powers ourselves. Many of us; however, were fortunate that life gave us the opportunity to train with truly amazing and highly accomplished Masters.

In the early to mid-1990's, I was living with my amazing wife Eileen in Augusta, Georgia. teaching Tai Chi and some Kung Fu. In one of the popular martial arts magazines of the time, I read the story of renowned Master, Henry Poo Yee. Master Yee had formed a new branch of the Southern Praying Mantis lineage which he called Chinese Kung Fu Academy (CKFA). Master Yee was living in Houston, Texas, so I would not be able to train with him on a regular basis. However, I thought to myself, if he had a student teaching in Georgia, or South Carolina, I might be able to train with that teacher. Amazingly, the author of the article, Sifu Jeff Larson, lived in Atlanta, so I called. We had a good conversation, but he informed me that he had recently returned to college full-time, was working part-time, teaching part-time and was married. He simply didn't have the time for another private student.

He said the Atlanta branch of CKFA was run by Sifu Peter Gouldburne. He gave me the schedule for the school, but I knew it wouldn't work as I needed to train on weekends, and I preferred to train privately. Also, something inside me told me that I was meant to train with him, so I called Master Yee in Texas. After I shared my lineage with Master Yee, and informed him I was teaching Tai Chi, he mentioned that he would speak with Jeffery (that is what he called Sifu Jeff) and ask if he could arrange time in his schedule to teach me.

To my surprise and delight, I received a call from Sifu Jeff, he said he had spoken with Master Yee and that he would make time in his schedule to teach me. I was ecstatic. Once I began training with Sifu Jeff, he said, "There are only two words you need to know in order to learn Kung Fu; 'Yes,' and 'Sifu.'- Yes Sifu! He told me that when Master Yee called and asked him to train me, "Yes Sifu" was the *only* response he could give. I do not believe that this level of respect exists as broadly today as it did back then.

Eileen and I drove from Augusta to Atlanta on a sunny summer day. When we arrived at Sifu Jeff's home he invited us in, introduced us to his lovely wife, Maura, and lead us into his office. Sifu Jeff said he liked to interview private students before he began teaching them. He wanted to understand their motivation, learn where their heart was and how they intended to use the Kung Fu he would teach them.

While I appreciate such talk, I am much more a man of action, this was made evident when Sifu Jeff began calling me Lei Kwai, from the story of the *Three Kingdoms*. Lei Kwai was famous for stripping naked and running headlong into battle, axes in hand, while screaming at the top of his lungs. I happily admit that does sound like me! We had been sitting and talking in Sifu Jeff's office for about twenty minutes when, to my delight, Sifu Jeff said, "It will be much easier to show you then to tell you, let's step outside." That was music to my ears.

Sifu's alter was located in his office, and he turned to bow and backed out whenever he left the room. Respectfully, we did the same and I turned to my wife Eileen and said with great confidence, "I am so going to drop this guy." This is the story of The Bending House (not about this particular day) but let me say this - I did not "drop this guy" as I so confidently believed I would. Instead, I got to experience Praying Mantis Kung Fu and I became - his student.

I have long believed that the great feats spoken of in Kung Fu lore are, or could be, true. I admit that I held out hope of witnessing a feat of some kind at some point in my life, but I never truly believed that I would be personally involved in one. My interest was rooted deeply in Tai Chi and Kung Fu, I loved the spring-like movement, the flow, the exploding and vibrating power these styles possess. However, Sifu Jeff kept talking about Qigong (chee gung). He said it was, in the words of Master Yee, "the fire inside of the Kung Fu."

Sifu Jeff was precise in his teaching. Whenever he taught something that was not exactly as he learned it, he would say, "these are not Sifu's words," or, "my interpretation of this movement is…" He continued to talk about Qigong, and I believe he wanted to prepare me; he was quietly planning to teach me Chi Kung as well as Kung Fu. But I was not always so patient in those days and I must have had enough of always hearing about Qigong, so one day I asked Sifu to show me this Qi power, this "fire inside the Kung Fu."

He explained that it not that sort of thing, instead, it is like a river - an energy that existed within and not some feat of power to display, like some trick pony. But I persisted. I did not let up. I begged him to show me a little something, to let me feel this Qi power. I told Sifu Jeff I would hold a phone book against my chest to absorb the power and prevent any possible injury.

Finally, Sifu Jeff agreed. I retrieved a phone book from inside the house and went out on the deck so I could finally see what this Qigong energy was all about. I had already trained for years with highly respected Tai Chi and Kung Fu Masters. I'd had the honor of feeling their energy during push hands, as well as other training techniques, so I believed there was no way he could move me off my stance.

First, Sifu Jeff showed me what he was about to do. He showed me how he would cup his hand, coil his wrist, coil his ankle, and lift his heal and then drop them all in unison as his palm released into the phone book. Fine. I thought this was more detailed than I imagined, and way more detail than I had patience for, but it was sort of what I thought it might be. Sifu Jeff explained that he didn't really like to do such displays, parlor tricks or pony shows as he called them, but that he would accommodate me *"this once."* He used to tell us, "My Qigong is like a soft breeze. Sifu's Qigong (Master Yee's) is like a hurricane."

I took my stance, right knee bent and turned in at a slight angle, hips, and shoulders straight forward, left leg bent and positioned behind me like a strut. I held the 3-inch phone book squarely on my chest, completely confident that I could absorb this little "pop" with ease. In fact, I was starting to feel a little sorry for this guy. After all, he'd spent all this time training Qigong, repeating frequently how Master Yee told him it was "the fire" inside of the Kung Fu and along comes this wise guy Kung Fu/Tai Chi Teacher from Augusta, about to absorb his little "palm pop," dousing the flame of his fancy little Qigong and its mythical power. I braced myself, for the little energy I believed was coming. Sifu Jeff cupped his palm, coiled his wrist and ankle like he said he would. Circling his elbow, he twisted and coiled his body, and, in a flash, he dropped his heel and released his palm into the phone book, and into my body.

Suddenly, everything changed. I don't remember feeling his palm "popping" into the phone book. Instead, there was a low, resounding sort of "poom" as his heel hit the deck in perfect timing with his palm release. And then it happened. My whole world went immediately into slow motion. I felt my body go airborne, and a strange sense of being aware of everything at the same time came over me. I know it sounds impossible, but as I reflect on the event, I feel like I was watching it happen from multiple points of view outside of myself, while also viewing it from within my body.

The distance from our location on the deck to the back wall of the house was about five or six feet. That is how far I traveled, through the air, before my body hit the house. This is where the world of slow motion truly took hold. As the full weight of my body hit the wall, I looked to my right to the edge of the house and watched as the wall began to bend inward with my weight. I felt myself sinking into it and I gazed with amazement as I saw the edge of the house disappearing the further I sank into the building.

Once the edge of the house disappeared from my vision, time seemed to stop completely. Everything seemed to go quiet, slow motion went into "no motion", time just froze. Then, as quickly as I was lifted into the air and was flying towards the wall, the house decided it had enough of me, and it sprang back into the solid form it once was, and I was again in flight, this time back in the direction of Sifu Jeff.

My flight from the wall was similar in distance to my flight to the wall, and I felt like I was at least a foot and a half off the ground, suddenly my feet landed on the deck in a soft, seemingly practiced sort of landing. As I landed on the deck, Sifu Jeff's left palm covered my chest and stopped my forward movement and his right hand, the one that had sent me into flight, was an inch in front of my face. It was coiled, pinky, ring finger and thumb were bend inward as if he was holding a ball with just those three digits. His middle finger was slightly bent, and his index finger was bent, pointing skyward and resting slightly against his middle finger. His hand had taken on the strange appearance of something lethal, of something I had never seen before.

I hope you will believe me when I tell you this - I see that vision as clearly today (more than 25 years later), as I did the moment it happened. The memory remains *that clear.*

With my hands now up in front of me and Sifu Jeff's left palm against my chest, I looked into his face with a sense awe and near disbelief. I will never forget the look on his face. It was a look that seemed to say, happy now? Actually, I was happy, in fact I was *very, very happy.* I knew from the moment that I left the ground that I was experiencing was something truly unique. At last, I thought to myself, at least some of the stories I've heard over all of these years are actually true.

After our class concluded that day, we returned inside the house to his office to discuss what we trained and to plan our next series of classes. When we entered his office, and I don't know why it never occurred to me before then, we looked to his alter on the East facing wall, the same wall that I hit from outside the house.

Sifu Jeff immediately walked over to the alter, which was in disarray, the ash pot that he placed the incense in, the bowl of oranges, the teacups and chop sticks—all of it was either knocked over or had fallen to the floor. Within a few minutes Sifu Jeff had the alter again in its original condition. He had lit incense, spoke silently to the Masters, and presented the incense which was now burning in the pot. Sifu didn't want me to help and had asked me to have a seat while he cleaned things up and restored the alter to its proper condition. As I watched, the same thought kept repeating in my head, "that really happened, that… really…happened!" As I drove home to Augusta that day, I clearly knew that something truly profound had happened, but I didn't know how to qualify it. I also knew that I may never experience something like that again.

In the years that followed, when Sifu Jeff taught me that hand position, he explained that as Masters developed their Qigong, their hand position would evolve from all fingers together to bent pinky and ringer finger and thumb with middle finger half bend with the slightly bent index finger leaning against the middle finger and appearing as if it was poised to pierce an opponent's body. He said he did not intentionally hold his hand that way, but that in that moment, it simply took on the shape once he dropped his palm into the phone book.

Sifu Jeff explained that when the index finger filled with Qi, it was referred to as "The Qi Needle." He explained that only the highest-level Masters ever separated the index finger from the middle finger and that doing so signaled to a potential opponent that they had this kind of (high level) Qigong. This was body piercing Chi energy. Master Yee said that when an opponent saw the Qi Needle, they would bow in respect and concede the impending fight or confrontation. This implies that only those who possessed such energy and displayed the Chi Needle, actually possessed the ability to use it. A Martial Artist of high degree has respect for tradition, ritual, and beliefs; thus, they would not display the symbolism of skills or abilities they did not possess.

To this day, any time I bring up this event or ask Sifu Jeff what skills or abilities he possesses, he simply states he had a Great Sifu and he is fortunate to train this Art. He never claims to possess any powerful or even unusual abilities. Saying this, it reminds me of another of Sifu Jeff's sayings, and he has many. "Those who know the most. say the least." Of course, he never once used that saying in reference to himself.

I have shared this story, on occasion, with my own students, and Eileen and I have spoken of it often. But until now, neither Sifu Jeff nor I have ever put that story into print. I did start training Qigong with Sifu Jeff after that—I mean, who wouldn't, right? I can say that there have been times, especially when training the Kung Fu immediately after training the Qigong, that I have felt a strong sense of internal power, a feeling of energy I never knew before, especially in my forearms. I would think to myself when the energy was especially present, "if I was ever going to try putting my fist through a wall, this was the time." Though I never did put my fist through a wall, I believe that this is the seed of what Sifu Jeff spoke of when quoting Grand Master Yee, "Qigong is the fire inside the Kung Fu."

I continue to train the early levels of Qigong on a daily basis, Sifu Jeff was very insistent about that (especially in the first 100 days) and I believe that my health is maintained largely due to the energy, and practice, of the Qigong. I still teach Tai Chi, Kung Fu, and Qigong on my country property in the woods of South Carolina just across the river from Augusta.

I mentioned to Sifu Jeff that I wanted to share "The Story of the Bending House" believing it would be a great addition to his revised book originally titled "Ancient Wisdom for Changing Times (The Master's Gift to the World), now called "The Power of Qigong" He said that it sounded like a good idea, especially since the book was about Grand Master Yee's Qigong and we had never shared the story publicly before. Sifu Jeff has now published the story on *ezine.com* after numerous rejections from Martial Arts publications. If we tell this story,

Sifu Jeff said, we should also mention two other things, which, though not directly related, do have a relationship to the story.

First, "The Greatest Warrior Wins Without a Battle." Sifu Jeff liked this saying and he said that Grand Master Yee liked it too and used it often. It implies that fighting should not be the first option, or even the second, perhaps, even the last option. This does not mean, Sifu Jeff would say, that you don't sometimes have to take immediate action or use your skill with little or no notice, but it does imply that when you can, it is better to settle differences without inflicting harm. Sifu Jeff said to me, in relation to my flying through the air – *that's the kind of power that the Qigong can generate, so we must be especially careful about ever using it against someone.*

Next, Sifu Jeff said he was going to allow me to use a word, more of a term really, which we almost never mention: Sun Gung. Sifu Jeff explains that "Sun Gung" is the name given to a unique kind of power and that there is no specific training related to this mysterious power. All Sifu Jeff would ever say about Sun Gung is that his Sifu, Grand Master Yee explained that unlike Ging or Qi, this energy was related to the three pillars of character, and that no one possessed it in a personal way.

The Grand Master said that the best one could do was to be a diligent student, to respect the System and the Masters, to be kind, compassionate and pure of heart. If one does all these things, Sifu Jeff said, perhaps one day you will experience *the presence* of very high level Qigong and that if you do you must understand that what you are experiencing is coming "through you, not from you." I thought about that for some time and concluded that he was ever-so-slightly suggesting *that perhaps, it was not "him" - that hit me".* That was it, now, I understood.

Sifu Jeff once shared the story of having lunch with the great Ving Tsun Master Moi Yat who is the Closing Hand Disciple (the last disciple) of the Great Ving Tsun Master, Ip Man. Ving Tsun is said to be the root, the origin of Wing Chun. Moi Yat had come with his top student (Miguel) to Atlanta to do a Ving Tsun Workshop. Sifu Jeff attended at the invitation of Sifu Cecil Sia Pao and Sifu Cooper. After the workshop, Sifu Jeff was invited to have lunch with the Master and his students. As he tells the story, he was seated directly across the table from Master

Moi Yat. At one point there was a break in the conversation and Master Moi Yat looked directly at Sifu Jeff and uttered words neither Sifu Jeff, nor anyone else at the table had expected, "You know Sun Gung," the Master said, half as a statement of fact, and half as a question. The table went silent as Sifu Jeff slowly looked up and over at Master Moi, and said, "My Sifu, Grand Master Yee has mentioned it, he has informed me about the pillars that must be in place for Sun Gung to come, but I would not say that I 'know' Sun Gung." Master Moi paused for a moment as a half-smile appeared on his face, he lifted his right hand, and as he did, it took the shape of the Qi Needle "You…. you know Sun Gung," Master Moi said shaking his hand with his index finger pointing at Sifu Jeff.

Sifu Jeff looked with respect at Master Moi and nodded in a bowing motion signaling respect, he never answered directly. Sifu Jeff said it would have been disrespectful to do anything else. The conversation at the table soon moved on to other matters. Perhaps, Sifu Jeff would say later, perhaps Master Moi Yat saw, or knew something about me that I did not know of could not see, myself. Regardless, Sifu Jeff would say, "it was an honor for such a great Master to simply talk to me. When he said what he did about Sun Gung, I was incredibly honored not just for myself but more for my Sifu, Grand Master Yee, because, if I possessed even a hint of potential related to Sun Gung, it was due *entirely to his efforts and training.*"

Thoughts from Sifu Tony Fabriguze
Written by Sifu Jeff Larson
Edited by Sifu Robyn Mathews-Lingen

Chapter 14

QUOTES FROM: HEALTH EXPERTS, OUR STUDENTS, ORGANIZATIONS AND CORPORATE CLIENTS

We have decided to relocate this chapter to our website "FloatingMonk.com"

Please visit us there to hear from our students and others in their own words.

Thank You.

Chapter 15

VISION AND OUTREACH: FROM THE ANCIENT WORLD TO THE MODERN DAY

From a general public perspective, Qigong is still relatively unknown (but that is slowly changing) Our hope in writing this book is to provide a simple, clear, and understandable explanation of Qigong, where it came from, why there are different types, and how it can benefit people.

The vision for Floating Monk is to provide Qigong Information, Education, and Training to the General Public, Businesses, and Organizations of all kinds. Qigong is our passion. We are convinced that Qigong can bring significant Physical, Mental, and even Spiritual benefits to those who practice it

Ancient Traditions

The ancient traditions are an intriguing aspect of Qigong. In our workshops, students have always shown great enthusiasm for learning about and discussing the Ancient Traditions. The Unspoken Codes and Who's Your Sifu are two important aspects of the ancient traditions (which we address in this book). The codes provide anyone interested in learning Qigong with a way to qualify potential programs and instructors, and to help potential students understand what qualities and certifications a potential teacher should possess.

Discussing the Unspoken Codes and other Taoist and Buddhist principles can help the reader to understand the values and principles of the Ancient Ways. As we discuss learning, understanding, and applying ancient wisdom, we believe it is important to know where the wisdom came from and why it is revered.

Floating Monk's Outreach Program

Our outreach program provides information, education, and training related to Qigong, we hope to serve as an information source for Qigong related Health and Wellness Programs in our communities and throughout the world.

Wellness

Wellness is the central focus of all Floating Monk programs, Wellness of Spirit, of Mind, and Body. Our Sitting, Standing, and Stretching Qigong programs address each of these important areas, and assist practitioners toward achieving the vision and goals they have for their own lives.

Our Website

After a brief time away, to update our programs, incorporate new findings, and integrate student "favorites", we are reactivating our website "FloatingMonk.com"

We will provide detailed information about our Qigong, Coaching and Wellness focused Training programs. We will also provide Training DVDs, Downloads, and other materials, including detailed written material to better understand and benefit from our training programs.

Classes and Workshops

Information about our Workshops will be available on our website. Workshops are currently being envisioned as ongoing events in Minneapolis/St Paul Minnesota and Atlanta/Roswell, Georgia, with plans for other U.S. Canadian, and European Cities in the future.

It is our desire to make our programs available to everyone, regardless of economic status. To achieve this, every workshop we teach will reserve places for individuals who may be economically disadvantaged. Sifu Robyn and Sifu Tim are especially interested in and will lead our efforts this area. They will help us, as an organization, to ensure that whoever wishes to learn our programs has the opportunity to do so.

Other Programs

Our website will provide links to other programs we support, such as those offered at the Ahemki Center in Roswell, Georgia, by Sifu Dr. Mark Armstrong (find out more about Dr. Mark's programs at <u>www. Ahimki.net</u>) as well as other, worthy endeavors.

To Complement or Enhance the Qigong Experience

We are also at work to provide links to other sites which can benefit practitioners of our programs and Qigong practitioners in general. In brief, we wish to make items available on our website which we believe can *enhance or complement health, wellness, and the overall Qigong experience.*

Sincerely
Sifu Jeff Larson

Sifu Jeff, assisted by a number of his Sifu's and Amazing Administrative Staff manage all the training programs offered by Floating Monk. This includes Workshops, multi-week Programs for those just beginning Qigong, as well as Advanced and Instructor Training Programs and Workshops. Sifu Jeff, and other Qualified Instructors, frequently travel to assist Individuals, Groups and Organizations seeking the benefit of the Floating Monk programs. To contact Sifu Jeff see the list at the end of the book.

For More Information

We welcome you to visit our website "FloatingMonk.com" for detailed information about our various programs and services. *We look forward to being of service.*

Chapter 16

BIOGRAPHIES

Sifu Jeff Larson

I grew up in small towns in Southern Minnesota. I attended Catholic grade school in Wabasha and Waseca, and public school in Lake City, where I graduated high school. For a couple of years during high school, our family moved to a suburb of Rockford, Illinois called Loves Park where I attended Harlem High School. I was the fourth of what would become thirteen children. My early memories of family life in those small towns is a loving one. Though we were lower middle class, we were close, we were loved, and life was good. We had loving Parents, Grand Parents and Relatives. At times our small-town life seemed almost like a Norman Rockwell painting.

I was interested in Martial Arts from a young age and was a big fan of the television show Kung Fu with David Carradine, and a big fan of Bruce Lee. I took my first classes, in Tae Kwoon Do while in Rockford. The School was close to the restaurant my father owned (and where I worked) I earned my yellow stripe but progressed no further before we moved back to Lake City, MN during my senior year of High School.

When I moved to Minneapolis following high school, I began visiting Kung Fu schools. I settled on a system called Southern Praying Mantis. That was almost forty years ago, and I am still involved with that system. After seven years in the system, I moved to Atlanta, GA. When I announced to my teacher that I would be moving to Atlanta, I was told, not asked, that I would be teaching once I got there.

Fate

Once I got settled in Atlanta, I began teaching individual, private students, next I began offering self-defense workshops. My first groups of students were waitresses from the restaurant where I worked, as well as their sisters and friends. Soon, a number of cooks, dish washers and others wanted to learn. By 1987 I had a room at a boxing gym (only a mile or so from the restaurant) dedicated to Kung Fu; I even sublet the space to another teacher on days when I wasn't teaching. One day a student came in for a private class holding a flyer for Kung Fu classes just a mile or so from where I was located. Competition from other schools is not unusual, what was unusual was that the system being advertised was the same one I was teaching. To my knowledge, I was the only person in the South-East teaching this type of Kung Fu, so I was intrigued and went to meet the teacher.

Within a few minutes of introducing myself and sitting down to talk with the instructor, I realized that I was in way over my head. I did not know it when I came into the school, but I was in the presence of a Master. I informed my students of the meeting and within a few weeks I closed my school at the boxing gym, and we all went to train with the Master who took me on as his assistant instructor.

Looking Back

I've reflected back on at that day many times over the years and considered everything that had to take place for that meeting to occur. Some people believe in fate, destiny, and serendipity, and others do not. For my part, I believe that my move to Atlanta was predestined. I believe that I was meant to go to Atlanta to meet the Master, Grand Master Yee.

Grand Master Yee taught me amazing things about the Kung Fu of Praying Mantis. He also taught me that the system had two parts, besides the Kung Fu there was also Qigong. While I loved the Kung Fu, I became more and more interested in the Qigong. My passion for Qigong and dedication to the system and the Master changed the course of my life. It is this dedication that's driven me for the past thirty years. My faith and conviction to Qigong is what pushed me to seek the Master's permission to show this Qigong to the world. That conviction was the driving force in developing Floating Monk (aka Chi for Health) Qigong. This passion was the fuel which sustained me over the course of many years as I wrote down, developed, taught, deconstructed, and reconstructed the programs.

As in any journey of this nature, there were sacrifices to be made. The pressure and demands of choosing this path can and did test my dedication and it has humbled me repeatedly in the process. Over these many years, there were several times when I wanted to walk away; I felt that the demands were too great and the price too steep to continue. On three occasions I went broke and on one occasion had to declare bankruptcy, but still I persisted. Sometimes in life, something grips you so deeply, attaches itself so completely that there is no way to separate yourself from it. When, and if, that happens, it is as if you have no choice, as if fate has found you and the ship has set sail. The destination remains unknown, but the course is set, there is no going back.

Getting Close to the Flame

In Qigong and Kung Fu, we refer to the opportunity to train with the Master as standing close to the flame. The Master is the living body and soul of the system, and very few people have the opportunity to train with a Master directly, especially for an extended period of time. This principle of standing close to the flame can apply to other areas of life as well, such as; sports, business, medicine, entertainment, working with a great chef, or in any number of other fields. If you have the opportunity in your life to stand close to the flame, to feel the pulse, energy, or essence of the knowledge you seek, do so, and savor the experience for it may never come again.

Train at the School, Learn at the Table

Train at the School, Learn at the Table is a term we often refer to in our system. In the school, as one imagines, the training is constant, it is physically and mentally demanding, and performed under the watchful eye of the Master. In the school, much of the talk is about the forms and techniques that various groups are practicing based on their level; there is not much time for conversation about anything except the training.

Once the evening of training is done, the Master often goes out to eat. If you are lucky, the Master may invite you to join him for dinner. Once you have been to dinner with the Master, you realize that those discussions are where the real education takes place. It is there at the table that you learn about the history of the system, hear the stories of long ago, learn about the skills of the Masters that preceded the current Master, and if the opportunity presents itself, you may even be allowed to ask questions. We make a point here about being allowed to ask questions because we often joke (but are actually serious) that there are only two words you need to know to learn Kung Fu and they are: "Yes, Sifu." In short, you keep your mouth shut, you do exactly what the Master says and if you ever do reply the only words you say are "yes Sifu."

The more often you are allowed to dine with the Master, the luckier you are. If you have been at the table for many years, you begin to hear the stories retold, often more than once, and this is no small blessing. In hearing the stories retold, you hear parts you had forgotten or perhaps missed on the first, second, or tenth telling. After hearing the stories told a couple of times (due to new people being invited to the table) you had a pretty good grasp of them. I was very fortunate when I closed my school and came with my students to train under the Master, as he allowed me to be his assistant instructor. This position allowed me to join the Master almost every evening for dinner. I now tell my students the stories which the Master told me all those years ago and have written this book, it part to preserve these stories for future students.

Our First International Tournament

In the autumn of 1991, Grand Master Yee and I attended an International Martial Arts tournament in Houston, Texas. I went to compete, and the Master went to teach workshops and see old friends. I competed in the Qigong/Internal Arts competition as well as the Southern Kung Fu Division. When you complete your routine, you salute and stand at attention awaiting your score. As I finished my Southern Kung Fu program, I could see the judges in the center and far corners of the ring looking at one other. I noticed the same thing occurring with the corner judges to my left and right. They appeared to come to agreements and flipped the numbers on their cards, I soon saw the scores as 9.9 and 9.8 scores appearing from the five judges. I knew I was near the top. One by one the other competitors entered and exited the ring. As soon as the competition was finished, the scores were announced. At the very first tournament that Grand Master Yee's Qigong and Kung Fu were seen; we won the gold medal!

I ran upstairs and waited for Sifu to notice me in the room where he was teaching a workshop. When I told him that I'd won the gold medal it was one of the proudest moments of my life. Although I was happy for myself, I was even happier for my Sifu as the gold medal was a clear statement of what the other Masters thought of Sifu's Qigong and Kung Fu. Sifu left Atlanta and moved to Houston a few months after the tournament. The following year, 1992, I attended the same tournament, this time held in Orlando, Florida. I went with students Sapir Tal, now Sifu Sapir Tal who is living and teaching in Israel, and Luis Cardozo, now living in Uruguay. I was extremely pleased with the results as each of them left the competition with gold and silver medals.

Before returning to college a few years later, I competed in a South-East regional tournament with other members of the Atlanta Branch School lead by Sifu Peter Goulburne and assistant instructors John Hall and Jonathan Gass. Once again, the Master's Qigong took home the gold medal and every member of the Atlanta School left the tournament with two or three medals. Peter took the helm of the Atlanta Branch School just before the tournament, and I turned to teaching private students while attending college full-time and working part-time. That was over thirty years ago. It is amazing how time flies.

After competing My BA in Finance in 1999, I began a new career in financial services. In March of 2011, I completed my MBA and now spend my time in two worlds: Financial Services and Qigong/Kung Fu.

Sifu Tony Fabriguzie

Sifu Tony Fabriguze (Augusta, GA.)

My name is Sifu Tony Fabriguze. I met and began training with

Sifu Jeff Larson in the summer of 1996. Through Sifu Jeff I came to meet and train with Grand Master Henry Poo Yee. It was during this time that my views and understanding of Kung Fu and Qigong took a leap forward. I still look at this period with incredible fondness and it continues to impact my training to this day.

I was born in Texas and lived there for the early years of my life. Grand Master Yee moved to Houston, TX in 1991, and during one of Grand Masters Yee's Annual Student Reunions, Sifu Jeff and I traveled outside of Houston to visit my Mother and brother who lived there at that time. I have lived in Georgia and South Carolina (with my wife Eileen) since the 1990's and consider this area of the country my home.

I am appreciative to Sifu Jeff for the opportunity of adding my history to this book and this history, the history of Tong Long Pai, Grand Master Yee's: Chinese Kung Fu Academy U.S.A. and his Ting Sing Qigong (aka Chi Kung) program. Finally, I am pleased that Grand Master Yee included me (in a discussion with he and Sifu Jeff) regarding the Masters permission to create "The Yee Gar Kung Fu System" to carry on the memory of our Great Teacher by preserving specific aspects of the Kung Fu that our great teacher gave to us.

My Kung Fu brother and mentor Sifu Jeff told me that one the reason he wished me to share my information and history was to let the interested public know that I am here in South Carolina (just across the river from Augusta, GA.) And that I am offering/teaching classes on a weekly basis. It has long been said (by Martial Artists) that some of the best Kung Fu is found in some of the most unlikely places. Sifu Jeff believes that my house on Silver Fox Court in Clarks Hill, SC is one of those places. Here is my story.

My Journey in Martial Arts:

1974: I started training 7 Star Praying Mantis under Sifu Ho Sing Fat. I trained with Sifu Fat for 10 years until his death in 1984. My favorite forms were mantis out of the Cave and Mantis steals the peach.

1984: I began training with my Kung Fu uncle Sifu Chan Poi of the Wah Lum Praying Mantis Tradition. I trained for seven years with Sifu Poi until I injured my leg. For the next few years I took a job which had me traveling the United States. In 1994 I landed in the Georgia/South Carolina area, were I settled down and stayed. My favorite forms were Wah Lum Kwan Doa and Lohan form.

1994 to Present: I trained Yang's Tai Chi under Sifu Lam Kwong Wing with a lot of input from Sifu Yang Jwing Ming, whom I consider a friend and mentor. I trained in Tai Chi Chuan from 1994 to present and I am a Certified Instructor of Yang's Tai Chi Chuan. My favorite forms are Yang Style long form and Yang Style Broadsword.

1996: I met and trained with my older brother and mentor Tai Siheng and Sifu: Jeff Larson for my first three years in Jook Lum Ji Tong Long Pai Southern Praying Mantis in preparation for our Master Henry Poo Yee's personal training and teaching.

1997: Completed my 1st Level of training in Southern Praying Mantis under Sifu Jeff Larson's care.

1998: Completed my 2nd Level of training in Southern Praying Mantis under Sifu Jeff's careful and very watchful eye.

1999: Completed my 3rd Level of training under Sifu Larson as well as Sifu Yee's care and guidance.

2001: Completed my 4th Level of training in Southern Praying Mantis under Grand Master Yee and Sifu Jeff Larson. I was promoted to the Senior Council and given permission to open a school under the guidance of Sifu Yee.

2004: Promoted to Full Instructor as well as private student of Sifu Yee as well as being adopted as his stepson. I still remember his loving and thoughtful words that day "Since I am your father now...you must listen and do what I tell you."

In the early 1990's Sifu Jeff was given permission by Grand Master Yee to form a New Branch School to teach the Qigong which the Grand Master permitted him to teach to the Public for the first time in the Systems History. This was a truly amazing honor. Sifu Jeff called this new branch: Floating Monk Qigong.

Then, in 2004: Sifu Jeff and Sifu Tony Fabriguze are given permission and commissioned to start a New Branch Linage of Southern Mantis *under the watchful eye of Grand Master Yee.* After Grand Master Yee honored us with this opportunity, I mentioned to Sifu Jeff that I would like to call the new Kung Fu branch "Yee Gar" (aka Yee Style Hand) in reference to and honor of Grand Master Yee's family name.

Sifu Jeff has honored me with the task of creating a detailed outline of the new system, including the levels of training, the specific exercises, the length of training and much more. With the outline complete Sifu Jeff and I will work closely together on a variety of matters including Alter Design, Uniform and Logo design, Training Materials, Workshop formats, Website and more.

Additional Notes

January 2019: After many years of training and having received numerous medals, awards, and other accolades in tournaments, and demonstrations, classes and seminars, Sifu Tony Fabriguze was recognized for achievement in Tai Chi Chuan, Chi Kung, and Kung Fu (Southern Mantis) by Schucker Martial Arts Association as well as being made a "Lifetime Member in Good Standing by the same organization.

History and Accolades

1974 to Present; Sifu Tony Fabriguze has been training Qigong and Kung Fu for 44 years. He has trained both Hard and Soft Qigong, Empty Hand techniques as well as 18 traditional weapons.

Sifu Fabriguze has been published by The Senior Citizens Council on Aging and has taught at: Powerhouse Gyms East & West, Fountainhead Fitness, Curves, Ladies Only, Health Central, Augusta Senior Center, and Thompson Senior Center.

Sifu Fabriguze has been a featured guest at Books a Million, Barnes and Noble, as well as the Cable Network Show "50 Plus" and The Augusta Chronicle on numerous occasions. The Thompson Times and Big Toys for Big Boys.

Sifu Tony and his students were also featured guests for the 1996 Olympic Torch Relay.

For over 44 years Sifu Tony Fabriguze has gone above and beyond to promote and teach the beneficial aspects of Tai Chi, Qigong (Chi Kung) and Kung Fu so that people from all walks of life, all ages and socio-economic classes could experience and benefit from these amazing arts and incorporate those benefits into their lives, just as he has into his own life.

A few words from Sifu Jeff

Sifu Tony is one of my longest training and most qualified students. He achieved great things, including advanced levels of Kung Fu training with me and Grand Master Yee. Tony achieved his Sifu status with Floating Monk, and it was well deserved.

As Tony was working toward achieving teacher status (in this System, while living in Augusta, GA), he already had a following of dedicated students. Many of his students began with him to learn Tai Chi (Tony was already a Certified Tai Chi Sifu), they saw in Sifu Tony a high level of skill and a deep understanding for his art, that quality has remained with him all of these years.

Sifu Tony's Praying Mantis (CKFA) students were hard working, dedicated, and well trained. They soon became recognized as some of the best students in our Federation, both for their hard work and their ability to correctly and effectively perform the Kung Fu forms and exercises. (a credit to their teacher)

As anyone who has read "The Story of the Bending House" will recognize, Sifu Tony has a bit of a Wild Man in him. I nick-named Sifu Tony "Lei Kwai" after the wild man in the Chinese Classic "The Three Kingdoms." Lei Kwai was known for stripping off his clothes and running into battle with a battle ax in each hand, screaming to the top of his lungs. Except for the naked part (thank God) that pretty much summarizes Sifu Tony.

Sifu Tony is a dedicated person to the core of his being. There is nothing he won't do for a fellow Kung Fu Brother, or Sister, and no effort he won't go to if asked by his teachers. Sifu Tony is the guard at the gate, vigilant, trust-worthy, never wavering, and ever ready to do what is needed to safe-guard, and promote, the System. He is also a long time, trusted, and much appreciated friend.

Sifu Robyn Mathews-Lingen

Journey to Qigong

One of the greatest things about my purple Huffy, with its two-tone bucket saddle and Malibu handlebars, was the chrome fenders, which made it look so much more like my brother's Dragster. It took me everywhere I wasn't supposed to be, including the karate school in the strip mall across the highway.

The sneakiest way to get there was to cut through Jimmy Brandt's backyard to 10th Avenue where virtually no kids lived. The route protected me from the watchful eyes of parents and siblings, and the school cook who lived next door. It was an adventure I took on Saturday mornings – crossing lawns, busy streets, the sandlot hill to the frontage road, then over the bridge to the mall where I stood with my bike watching the boys rush from their fathers' Buicks to the open door of the karate school.

I had been in that studio, with its gleaming wood floor and rack of Black Belt magazines, and they had said "no," this was not a place for girls. The disappointment of it coursed through me for weeks as I stood on the sidewalk, angry and hurt and expecting to be invited in.

My father had said, "honey, you're a born athlete. Your day will come." And I believed him. But what I didn't understand was that although he championed my born-to-throw arm, other men sought to tamper the tomboy, to teach her a lesson about what it meant to be a girl.

In time, I swapped my Hannie Caulder poster for David Cassidy, and gave in to all thing's girl. I would go on to play and coach softball, but by the time Title Nine was in full swing, my father had died, and the orthopedic surgeon had said to wait 10 years, when arthroscopy would be the cure for my crumpled knee. There was no future for girls in sports anyway.

But where everyday folks squashed their neighborhood tomboys, Hollywood, Rock'n Roll and the Olympics began to lift them up. So, for every episode of abuse that had come my way, there was a woman on a stage who showed me how to cut through it. In time, I settled into college and career and Tuesday night softball. I fell in love and married, finding even deeper joy in our children.

It was easy to give everything of myself to my family. They opened my heart, steadied my mind, filled my soul. They lifted my father from the confines of my subconscious to surface of my being, so that I might become the best of him. But hanging out on the couch with toddlers and a pile of books made me flabby, and when running a single flight of stairs left me breathless, heart pounding, I made my way back to a karate school, unaware of the inner tumult that would rise up - and the healing that would follow.

I thought I understood the fear many women feel about studying a martial art. While I was always attracted to it, most women I knew instantly dismissed it; too difficult, too violent, too male, too time-consuming. But the doors were now open. Women were competing in the Olympics and in martial arts schools across the country. I had always played like a boy, but I was not prepared for the level of diffidence that would surface. Inside, I became as timid as a rabbit crossing an open field.

One third to one half of women, depending on the color of her skin, experience sexual assault. If they were young, the repugnance of it will fester. Indeed, they may grow to perfect the costumes of workers, wives and mothers, but all too often, these vestments conceal chasms of pain, depression, anxiety and grief. My own fissures had muddled my mind, broken my heart, shut down my body, deadened my soul. But very few knew that. Very few would look past my own costume of success to all that was missing underneath. Perhaps, for this reason, I always wore my full uniform to train, no matter how hot and humid the studio. While others came to class in t-shirts and shorts, I wore my black canvas gi at all times. It protected me on the outside from all that male sweat, and it protected me on the inside from all that self-doubt.

My green belt, soft and a little frayed, became the level in which I would pivot from learning my art, to understanding my art. For the first time, I had struggled to remember the forms. Lunges and kicks had challenged me, hand combinations felt inaccurate. And just as I had been taught as a little girl, I began to think that this was no place for me.

It is habitual. It is what brought me to the studio early on a steamy

September evening. I took the floor alone to run this form; forward, backward, in four winds, until it was embedded in muscle like mineral in soil. But on this day, something triggered memories of the man whose statutory violation of my young tomboy body had fractured my very being. Long dead, his ghost stood before me in the empty studio, teaching me a lesson, churning my fears, fueling self-doubt. And that is when, for the first time, rage surfaced. My imagination took over, and I ran the form around and through him until I had beaten him. Mind, body and breath coalesced. I had touched the art of it.

Years would pass before meeting Sifu Jeff Larson at a coffee shop with a mutual friend. Within the first few mocha sips, Sifu had become my teacher, and qigong had become my friend.

At my first lesson, I had expected to see the qigong we see everywhere - choreographed movements of mystery readily available on YouTube. When this was not the case, when I stood for an hour breathing into the most subtle motion, I felt confused. I couldn't see the power. I couldn't feel the energy. I didn't understand a single moment of it. "You're a born athlete," my dad had said. But apparently, qigong was not impressed by my athleticism, nor my degrees of black belt, and she kept her distance.

Some teachers tell you what to do. Others lead you to the shores of synthesis, and there, they can lead you to yourself. It wasn't magical, it wasn't revelatory, but in time I could feel how qigong weaves itself through and around the sinew of life. Today, it takes but a moment to feel the heat of qi when I step forward, take position. I am grateful to Sifu Jeff for bringing me to this place, where I can become a part of living qi, and find my best self.

Sifu Robyn Mathews-Lingen earned her Fifth Degree Black Belt in Shaolin Kenpo under the precise and gentle teaching of Professor David Meyer, Seventh Degree Black Belt and student of the late Great Grandmaster Ralph Castro. She became Sifu of Qigong under the wise guidance of Master Jeff Larson, Enter the Gate Disciple of Grandmaster Henry Poo Yee, Praying Mantis Kung Fu. She would not have accomplished either without the steadfast encouragement and loving support of her beloved partner and spouse, Ann; her courageous, insightful daughters, Emma and Claire; and her companion fur-teacher, Penny.

A few words from Sifu Jeff

I would like to add that Sifu Robyn is the only student of mine to train up to and beyond the Third Level of Floating Monk Qigong since 2012. This fact and my knowledge of her passion for this Qigong has led me to assign Sifu Robyn as the Lead Training Instructor for Floating Monk Qigong for the state of Minnesota, and beyond. In the future, I will very likely be assigning additional titles and roles to Sifu Robyn as it relates to her achievements and this position. I want it to be known that whatever title she assigns to herself, in an instructor related capacity, I trust that she will do with the well-being of Floating Monk in mind, and she has my full confidence and support.

I like and have complete confidence in Sifu Robyn, she is a good person with high moral character and I believe that she can and will achieve whatever goals she sets for herself. I envision Sifu Robyn working in many capacities, and perhaps many countries as we work to bring Floating Monk to a global audience. From our earliest days of training, Sifu Robyn's passion for her Martial Art, and for Floating Monk Qigong, were evident. She is passionate about giving back to her community and the larger world through teaching. I also know that Robyn is dedicated to teaching self-defense, and since Floating Monk is rooted in Kung Fu, I would like to see Floating Monk assist Sifu Robyn in her efforts to help young girls, women and others ward off anyone who would try to abuse them, robbing them and our community of their youth and innocence.

Sifu/Dr Mark Armstrong

Sifu/Dr Mark Armstrong's Biography, including his ideas of training with Sifu Jeff and working together to produce Floating Monk Qigong Training Workshops, can be found at our website "FloatingMonk.com" Please visit us there for Sifu/Dr Mark's amazing story

A few words from Sifu Jeff

Dr Mark was a very dedicated student. On a weekly basis, he drove to my studio in Midtown Atlanta from the Northern Suburbs, in all kinds of weather. He understood the principles quicker than many students due to the fact he was already a Certified Doctor of Chinese Medicine and Acupuncturist. Many people do not know it, but Dr Mark was my Reiki teacher (Master) and in the advanced stages of my training he invited me (and fellow Reiki students) to work with him in a clinical environment for many months. He would treat patients with various modalities and I, and my fellow Reiki students, would work on patients after his treatments. In addition, I would often instruct patients in Basic Qigong and we found this to be a wonderful compliment in their overall healing process.

Many years ago, I saw a vision of Dr Mark speaking and teaching (which included this Qigong) to a National / International Audience. I still believe that vision will come true and I hope to be there (as a part of the Floating Monk Team) to applaud his achievements and perhaps provide support to the Qigong part of his program.

Sifu Pascal Sellem

Pascal was born on 1970 in Paris, France to Jacky & Monique Sellem. He grew up in those early years in predominantly Jewish environment.

Pascal moved at the age of nine to the United States with his family. His parents opened a French restaurant in Birmingham, Alabama and for the next eight years they integrated into life in the U.S. and moreover, in the South.

As a teenager, he worked in his parents restaurant assisting Dad in the kitchen as young sous-chef and, when needed, helped out as a busboy or dishwasher. Pascal understood the importance of helping his family in their endeavors, and how his efforts played a part in his parents, and his family's success. After eight years in Alabama, the family moved to Sarasota, Florida for eighteen months before finally settling and making their home in Atlanta, Georgia.

In 1991 Pascal started school at a hairstyling college while apprenticing with his hairstylist uncle until 1994. In 1995 Pascal opened his first hair salon and has operated as an Independent Salon Owner and Stylist ever since.

In 2006 Pascal met Sifu Jeff Larson, he soon became a private student and quickly dedicated himself to Sifu Jeff's Qigong program and Martial Arts teachings. Over several years of one on one weekly lessons, and gradual advancement through Sifu Jeff's Teachers program, Pascal became a Certified Qigong Sifu.

Sifu Pascal also studied additional philosophies, such as The Tao, Kabbalah and an assortment of Eastern Philosophical and Spiritual teachings. Sifu Pascal credits these teachings with having a great influence in his day to day Qigong practice as well as his teaching style, which focuses on helping every student open up to and realize their fullest potential.

Sifu Pascal is committed to sharing everything he has learned with his students, friends, family, and others to make the world a better place. In Sifu Pascal's words "Mind, Body & Spirit are the essence of Qigong. "Breath leads to the key which unlocks the Holy Spirit which in turn communicates with God." Sifu Pascal

Sifu Pascal Sellem can be reached at 678-427-2963 or by email at scizzorhand@mac.com

A few words from Sifu Jeff

Pascal has been a very dedicated and determined student since the earliest days. He is someone who is a pleasure to teach and a joy to be around. He is a quick study and a diligent student. In addition to Sifu Pascal being a recognized and respected Master Stylist (in the French Method), Pascal has a passion for and an intuitive understanding of technology, which I believe can and will help us to promote and teach this Qigong. It is both my hope and my goal to work with Sifu Pascal to help design and develop web-based training and out-reach programs which Floating Monk can share throughout the World.

I have no doubt at all that Sifu Pascal will rise to the challenges and opportunities that await us and, that he will succeed in spectacular fashion. Sifu Pascal also possesses a unique talent in regard to language, he speaks fluent French. I strongly believe that with his language skills, and his natural ability and enthusiasm for speaking to and teaching in front of, groups of all sizes, he can help Floating Monk to expand Internationally.

He spent his early years in France, and I believe Floating Monk Qigong may provide the means for Sifu Pascal to return there as an accomplished, recognized Qigong Instructor. I am confident that his knowledge, ability, and passion for Qigong will translate both in his energy and language to bring Floating Monk Qigong to France, and perhaps Europe in general. I envision great things for Sifu Pascal.

Sifu Tim Hubachek

When I was a teenager still in Junior high school, I developed a love and passion for health, fitness, and nutrition. I gathered books, magazines, and any information I could find regarding these topics. I started training awfully hard with weights when I was 16 and was able to put on about 55 pounds of muscle during my four years of high school. My passion for working out soon transferred into wanting to assist others in their health and fitness journey. I went on to do 8 years in the Army as a Combat Engineer and volunteered myself to help the unit and individual soldiers improve their strength, endurance, and body composition to make them perform better on their fitness tests, in training and in combat. During this time, I got certified as a personal trainer and received a Bachelor's degree in Health Promotion and Wellness with a Fitness Leadership minor. For the last 7 years, I worked full time in the fitness industry. While most of my field experience has been in personal training, I have also branched into corporate wellness, health promotion, gym operations and other related categories to build diversity and strengths in many areas of health and fitness.

Since graduating college, I have lived in 3 different states, including Wisconsin, Florida and Minnesota gaining experience in the fitness world. I have trained and coached well into the hundreds of people but feel this is just the tip of the iceberg. After ETS, I moved to Tampa FL to begin a new life and adventure. Just a short 15 months after moving there, I was in a horrific motorcycle crash which was near fatal and completely debilitating. Due to the hand of God and skilled surgeons, I not only survived, but over a period of a painful and grueling 3 months in the hospital, was able to walk out, literally! But the battle was far from over. Over the next couple of years, I had 3 more corrective surgeries to my right knee and right arm. These allowed less pain and allowed me to continue gaining strength and mobility. During this time of recovery and rehab, I moved to the Minneapolis area to resume building my career and pursuing my goals. I originally took a job in personal training for Lifetime Fitness, but after 8 months there I accepted a position at Ameriprise Financial as a fitness specialist. It was at this location that I had the honor and privilege to meet Sifu Jeff. After knowing one another for about a year, we designed and implemented a self-defense workshop, open to all Ameriprise employees. The pilot class was highly successful, and we were able to teach basic and easily applicable fundamentals of self-defense to a very novice demographic.

While in the Army and for a three-year period after (2011-2015), I studied and practiced Taekwondo at a school in Wisconsin. By practicing an average of fifteen hours each week, I was able to become proficient quickly, attaining my 1st Degree Black belt after fifteen months, and my 2nd Degree after four years. However, due to the injuries sustained in the crash, my body could not continue the level of training necessary to reach higher ranks in Taekwondo. Shortly after my discontinuance from competitive Taekwondo is when I met Sifu Jeff.

Having a martial arts backgrounds triggered an immediate connection. Sifu Jeff, with much more experience and many more years teaching martial arts, deserved and received a high level of respect from me. Over time, our conversations regarding teaching and practicing martial arts led to the development of implementing a self-defense program at our work. Sifu Jeff and I successfully blended elements of Kung Fu, Floating Monk, Taekwondo, Krav Maga and Qi Gong, allowing the group to learn situational awareness, hand to hand and foot combative techniques, as well as the connection between mind, body and breath to deliver both presence and power.

In May of 2017, I was diagnosed with Stage III Melanoma, right after a large and painful mole appeared on my upper right chest. Dermatologist and general surgeons removed it as well as affected lymph nodes in right arm pit within a month. Thinking that was the end, I proceeded on with my life as usual, but had follow up scans and CT imaging every 3 months. In August of 2018, a scan detected that the cancer had spread to my liver and lungs at a very significant level. The oncology team recommended and stressed the need for chemotherapy to rid these areas effectively. Having some time to think about it, I began Chemo in Jan 2019 and did treatments every 3-4 weeks through September. The chemo was very effective at removing the cancer, at least from the neck down that is. An MRI in Oct showed an immense growth in my left frontal lobe. The radiology and oncology team determined it was a metastatic tumor, related to the previous cancer. The neurosurgeon team scheduled me for immediate extraction (Nov 12, 2019). After the tumor extraction, I took 2 months of medical leave to rest the body and brain and complete Gamma knife radiation, to really improve my odds of the cancer not returning to the brain.

During my battle with this cancer, Sifu Jeff trained and coached me on the art of Qi Gong. With this training, I further learned the importance and power of connecting the spiritual and mental dimensions to improve the physical and emotional realm. Coming from someone who has had significant health challenges and physical limitations, I truly realize the potential power of the Qi Gong art. Done correctly, one can experience the healing power of the breath, as well as channeled blood and energy flow. This art can be an extremely useful tool to help one eliminate or greatly reduce negative emotions and their associated side effects. It also has the potential ability to rid the body of toxins, inflammation, and free radicals. Perhaps we can all agree that these properties can benefit just about anyone! During my Level 1 certification in Qi Gong with Sifu Jeff, I experienced a release of many negative and pressing thoughts, feeling much less anxious and stressed than before the class. Personally, I believe we as humans are strongest when we connect with God the creator and the healing His Son brought for us on the cross. Recognizing Him as Lord will maximize the power and potential of Qi Gong, because Christ came to this earth to bring us eternal salvation. On the cross, He also bore all sickness infirmity and disease known to man, so that we would not have to. I choose to allow Him to take my burdens and use Qi Gong to connect more deeply to my faith and with who God says that I am.

My vision is to be able to reach, affect and impact thousands upon thousands of individuals seeking better physical and spiritual health, influenced by my testimony and personal journey to accomplish my life's goals and dreams through near-impossible odds. I personally feel that my purpose on earth is to use my second chance at life to come alongside others in a way that I couldn't have before – to relate, empathize and coach one along – through physical challenges, struggles and obstacles and still set out to accomplish the most they can, and the purpose God has set aside for them.

A few words from Sifu Jeff

I first met Sifu Tim while working at Ameriprise Financial Services, where Tim was a Trainer and Manager. I trained quietly on my own and observed, as is my style, I soon determined that he was very good at what he did. Over time conversations arose, often going for longer and longer periods especially where his military training or his Martial Arts experience were concerned.

Our discussions evolved into the idea of offering Simple, Immediately Effective and Easy to Remember (and repeat) Martial Arts techniques for novices. Tim took the lead and soon we had promotional material, a name for our program, and a schedule, we were off and running. Over the following Year, Sifu Tim and I taught numerous large classes of novices in 6 to 8-week workshop type formats. Both Sifu Tim and I are confident that many of those participants could (to this day) immediately and effectively deliver the techniques they learned, if confronted, and get away from a potentially harmful situation with minimal if any, harm to themselves.

In addition to the Floating Monk Qigong, I envision working again with Sifu Tim to develop programs similar to the ones we taught and to offer these programs via Workshops, Downloadable Self Learning programs and a wide assortment of Kung Fu/Qigong based Health and Wellness Programs. I know that Sifu Tim is dedicated to practicing and teaching Floating Monk Qigong and I firmly hope to have Sifu

Tim grow with Floating Monk and help us to bring this Qigong to an interested, benefit seeking audience across the globe.

I have complete trust in Sifu Tim, and I strongly believe that challenges he has faced, including multiple cancer treatments, have instilled in him a deeply empathetic, loving, focused desire to help others to both survive and grow as they go through similar struggles. Sifu Tim has a "no quit" quality to him This is evident is his work, in his faith and in his desire to help others.

I firmly believe that Sifu Tim brings all those qualities to Floating Monk and that together we can help people across the globe to live happier, healthier, longer, and more joyous lives.

Sifu David R Pease

Born In March of 1960, the fourth of nine siblings, life as I remember would be filled with hand-me-down toys, mischievous adventure, and mismatched socks. I recall the idealism and tragedy of the Kennedy era, my unbridled energy to a variety of sports and summers of fishing, hiking, and exploration growing up at our family cottage near Detroit Lakes MN, The sights and sound of a Rockwellian upbringing darkened only by the realities of drama and dysfunction that would finally usher in new chapters and the challenges as a blended family, we all faced.

It was a restaurant in the Twin Cities, where we both worked, that would bring about the friendship I have known these 40 past years with Sifu Jeff. Young, philosophical, and disciplined to his pursuit of poetry writing and martial arts. he was more naturally someone that I found resonated within my own views and by this would set a course that we have continued to share.

Though we would go on to evolve our interests through different professional and educational means, It is fair to say his influence has steadied my outlook on the Arts and Art of living in solid ways, but foremost it is his Qigong and the commitment to "Aging with Class" that continues to drive my goals for future accomplishment.

Here is a brief summary of my efforts across the years since Jeff and I first met.

I am 60 years and have been a Qigong practitioner since 2012 and a Certified Sifu March 2018

1978 -1983 Therapeutic massage therapist/ Chinese wand exercise instructor

1983-1995 Arthur Murray Dance Instructor And Owner of On 42nd Ballroom

1995 to present Retail Flooring/ Installations

Having an interest in and studies of human anatomy and movement I have always believed in proper breathing and stretching techniques. My experience and training with Sifu Jeff have resulted in my further belief these forms are wonderfully beneficial to stress management and to the proper function of our body systems in digestion and elimination. I encourage the practice of Qigong as early in life as possible but have found the benefits and ease of its routine makes for an ideal daily exercise at any age. Good Health to you all,

An insightful, informed, even philosophical view of life, combined with the vast river that is Qigong can help us to - As the Poet, Dylan Thomas states "Advance, for as long as forever is"

A few words from Sifu Jeff

David R, as he is known, is one of my oldest and dearest friends. We have seen each other through marriages and divorces, moves from state to state, various vocational changes and the maturation of our once (and forever) philosophical, poetic, and artistic view of the world and of life in general.

David has long had an ability to grasp and perform physical movement, whether in his years as a Dance Instructor, or as a Qigong Student. I have observed David's passion for the movement, the energy, and the benefit that Qigong delivers, both immediately and over time. I have enjoyed observing and being a part of David's growth as both a student and as a teacher.

I am confident that David will continue to grow in his understanding of Qigong and his abilities as an Instructor and I am glad to have him with me, and all of us (at Floating Monk) on this journey. I have a strong sense, and a deep hope, that David will evolve with Floating Monk as we work toward our goal of teaching in North and South America, Canada, France and across Europe. I look forward to having him at my side, and at our side (all of us with Floating Monk) as we step forward - into this great journey.

Christopher Larson (Future Sifu and Younger Brother of Sifu Jeff Larson)
U.S. National Level Competitive Skate Boarder, and Martial Artist

I grew up primarily in small towns in Southern Minnesota (Lake City and Winona) with brief excursions to Loves Park, IL and Royal Oak, MI when our family moved for job related reasons. I've felt the competitive drive from an early age, perhaps from being the youngest of 13 children and of seven boys. I began skateboarding at an early age. I evolved quickly and soon became good enough to compete at the National Level.

National Level Live Street Skating is an intense, physically demanding, highly competitive, and often dangerous sport. It was a sport I loved, and still love, for a number of reasons. Competitive skating afforded me the opportunity to travel throughout the U.S., to compete on a very high level to meet and learn from other skaters, and to push myself on a daily basis to be better than the day before.

As time passed the circumstances and demands of my life changed, I moved beyond Competitive Street Skating but my desire to continuously learn and grow remained in place. In my search for an activity or sport that I could learn and grow with, I found Martial Arts. Martial Arts offered me, as Skateboarding did, a freedom of expression, of self. It allowed me to choose what level I wanted to obtain, to practice, to perfect. I also love that with Martial Arts one can learn a technique and then practice it on their own.

My sense of self could remain intact and even enhanced through the practice of Martial Arts. It is a sport, a practice, a lifestyle where I can function, learn and grow on a long-term basis. I've found that through practice of the movements, both by myself and with practice partners, that Martial Arts gave me a deeper sense of both confidence and drive.

The feeling of practicing a Martial Art was different than feelings I experienced with Skateboarding, it provided a sense of awareness coupled with a quiet, calm feeling of both focus and relaxation.

Over the years I have had the opportunity train with three different, wonderful and giving Sensei's (a Karate based word for Teacher or Master) in both Wisconsin and Minnesota. In life, we tend to move through various phases of change, areas of focus, etc. Currently, I practice what I have learned on my own, often in the early morning, sometimes even late at night, but I do continue my practice. In the future, both near and distant, I plan to return to the Karate practices of recent years to achieve advanced belts and perhaps to even evolve to some level of teaching.

I also hope to have the opportunity to train with my Sifu/brother (Sifu Jeff, the author of this book) as I have long had an interest in the Kung Fu system he trained as well as the Qigong practice which is a part of that Art. I believe that training in Martial Arts provides a wide variety of benefits, I have personally experienced many of these benefits which is part of the reason I hope to teach; I would like to share these benefits with others and to help them experience these benefits in their bodies and their lives.

These are the benefits I have experienced and wish to share:

- Being involved with positive people as they develop new skills, they can use to protect themselves, their loved ones and their friends
- Learning a valuable Martial Art that instills and enhances in the practitioner's sense of drive. This quiet drive, this confidence permeates his or her spirit and flows into their personality, home life, career and community.
- From l-being. My brother (Sifu Jeff says) "Discipline begets discipline" and Martial Arts practice enhances the act of follow through in the school as well as in their life. Once a student achieves one level (sash or belt) they realize that; if they can achieve that level, they can achieve the next level and the one after that.

A few words from Sifu Jeff

While Chris and I have had numerous conversations about Qigong and various styles of Martial Art, he has yet to begin his formal training of this Qigong. While I may well be his primary Sifu, I am very pleased to know that we, as a system, now have many Qualified Instructors to assist in his training.

Chris is physically gifted in regard to various pursuits. In his early years Chris was an amazing skilled Break Dancer, I often marveled at his abilities. When he focused his attention on Street Style Skateboarding, he developed into an accomplished competitor and joined and competed in National Street Skating Demonstrations and Competitions across the U.S.

Currently we live in different cities (I am in Minneapolis and he lives almost two hours South, in Winona, MN), I trust, and believe that time and circumstance will eventually allow Chris to train this Qigong and that in time he will become a thoughtful, skilled, and highly accomplished, Qigong Instructor.

Chapter 17

CONCLUSION

History

One of the central themes throughout this book has been history. We have talked about the history of Qigong in general, the history of this system of Qigong, and of the Master of the system, Grand Master Henry Poo Yee, who has allowed us to share this information with you. We have discussed the idea of people being born into their time, or at a point in history when what they contribute has a potentially significant influence upon us as individuals, as a society, and as a human family.

History is the great educator. Poets, philosophers, painters, and musicians are all fond of history. Through their gifts of reflection in essays, poetry, painting, and song, we feel the pulse and power of our own lives and the feeling of community with the generations to which we belong.

It is difficult or even impossible to measure the influence of such individuals as Mahatma Gandhi, Martin Luther King Jr., John F. Kennedy, Wolfgang Amadeus Mozart, Handel, Christopher Marlowe, Vincent Van Gogh, Dylan Thomas, Robert Frost, Albert Einstein, and an endless list of others, until their lives are over and their influence is fully recognized.

Ancient Wisdom and Modern Life

The Qigong which the Grand Master has allowed us to show to the public could not have been timelier. The simplicity of the motions, and the easy, relaxed breathing techniques, allows the very young to the very old to learn and benefit from these programs. As the founders of the Floating Monk (Chi for Health) Qigong series of programs, we feel honored and extremely fortunate to be able to offer the world so great a gift at a time when its benefits are so needed.

By giving his permission, Grand Master Yee demonstrated what it means to be of service to others, and to reflect the light, wisdom, and knowledge of those who came before us. We believe that his lifelong efforts to teach, preserve, and advance his art and the CKFA system *will surely place his footprints upon the sands of time.*

We would like to finish this book with these words: Thank you for your interest in our book. We hope that the information we provided, and the stories we shared have been interesting, informative, and entertaining, but most of all, we hope that you enjoyed what we've provided and feel that this information has brought value to your life. Please visit our web site for training materials, or attend a Workshop, multi-week Program or Private Class as it is our wish that *"You - personally experience the benefits of the Qigong we offer."*

Finally, ...
Perhaps all of us - in consideration of the many gifts we have to
offer one another and the world at large - were born into our time.
Floating Monk / Chi for Health

List of Instructors and Contact Information

Sifu Jeff Larson
Jefflarson333@gmail.com

Sifu Tony Fabriguzie
Aka: Lei Kwai (706) 831-7193

Sifu Robyn Mathews-Lingen
Dragoncrane.org (651) 260-0730

Sifu Dr Mark Armstrong
Mark.Armstrong@ahimki.net (770) 552-4242

Sifu Pascal Sellem
scizzorhand@mac.com (678) 427-2963

Sifu Tim Hubacek
Timhubacek@yahoo.com (715) 803-3690

Sifu David R Pease
David.R.Pease@yahoo.com

PGIL2021USA